Nurse-led Change and Development
in Clinical Practice

'Do not believe a word that I say until you have gone into the wards and proved it. There you will find your great book of instruction. I only pretend to supply a key, a glossary or an index to it. Use that book as one ought, and then, though in the end you and I may have the same knowledge it will not be because it has passed from my mind to yours, but, being gained by your own observation, ratified by your own proofs, and matured by your own thought, you will have it and hold it as your own independent possession.' Peter Mere Latham, 1789–1875

Nurse-led Change and Development in Clinical Practice

Loretta Bellman

PhD BSc (Hons) RN RCNT RNT Cert Ed
Independent Consultant and Senior Researcher
The Bayswater Institute, London

WHURR
PUBLISHERS

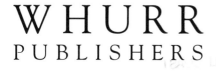

© 2003 Whurr Publishers Ltd
First published 2003 by
Whurr Publishers Ltd
19b Compton Terrace
London N1 2UN, England, and
325 Chestnut Street, Philadelphia PA 19106, USA

British Library Cataloguing in Publication Data
A catalogue record for this book is available from the
British Library.

ISBN 1 86156 337 X

Printed and bound in the UK by Athenaeum Press Ltd,
Gateshead, Tyne & Wear

Contents

Foreword

I am delighted to provide a foreword for this timely volume on nurse-led change and development. Nurses are no strangers to change and as such would be considered expert in its management. However, it is only now that nurses are beginning to succeed in terms of taking the change initiative and making real contributions to the shaping of health- and social-care policy and practice. Being a 'change agent', whether in clinical practice, education, management or research, is not an easy option. Having the appropriate skills, as well as the courage to stick one's 'tall poppy' head above the parapet is essential, not least because the opposition to what one is trying to achieve will come from many quarters, including (and this is often the most difficult to deal with) nurse colleagues.

An understanding of collaborative change processes as well as those that are disempowering are essential tools for change agents in nursing. Being at the leading edge of change can be exhilarating, career enhancing and make for intensive personal growth. However, it is worth remembering the playwright Tennessee Williams's cautionary words that 'high station in life is earned by the gallantry with which appalling experiences are survived with grace'. May this book actively enhance the gallantry and graciousness of its readership, as well as help to reduce the incidence of appalling experiences. May you all achieve the high station in life that you, as 'nurse change agents', so richly deserve.

Roswyn Hakesley-Brown
President, Royal College of Nursing 2002

Abbreviations

ALs	activities of living
CD	clinical director
DN	director of nursing
DSU	day surgery unit
NDU	nursing development unit
NUM	nurse unit manager
TM	theatre manager
TTO	medication to take out on discharge from hospital
WHO	World Health Organisation

Acknowledgements

How can I possibly do justice to all the people who, over many years, have influenced my thinking about being a nurse and nursing, which culminated in the research study and the writing of this book? These are the family members, friends, patients, supervisors, past students and library staff of the Royal College of Nursing and working colleagues (in practice, education, management and research) who have supported and challenged my ideas and working practices and continue to do so.

Although many people supported and contributed to the research in both hospitals, I could not have undertaken the studies without the co-researchers. Their trust in me, and their commitment to enhancing the quality of patient care, enabled me to facilitate the clinical change process. Their good humour and practical wisdom provided a positive force for exploring the status quo and innovative practice. Their consent to participate in the research included their wish to retain their anonymity.

I would also particularly wish to thank my research supervisor Graham Howes, who 'rescued' me, and the many people who have also 'lived' the study with me including my immediate family, Peter, Douglas and Bobbo The Bird. A special thank you also to Marion Newson, Mary Brown, Suzanne Graves, Kim Manley and Belinda Carson (she knows why!). I am indebted to Ruth Davies and Kate Dewar, who critically reviewed the text and provided me with untainted feedback. At Whurr Publishing I valued Jim McCarthy's 'light touch' and wealth of experience. I discovered the Collaborative Action Research Network (CARN) at a critical time in the research, and I continue to value the many members who contribute to my life-long learning and professional development.

Funding for the study came from the Royal College of Nursing Institute, the King's Fund and the University of Greenwich.

Introduction

'Even when we know where we are going, we still need to know how to get there.' (Cope 1981)

The approach to nurse-led change and development

How may nurses within current healthcare settings be enabled to develop, update and advance their knowledge and lead *patient-focused change and innovation in their field of practice? This book is for practitioners, practice educators, researchers, managers and colleagues who wish to explore a way of working, learning and researching together. Nurses in practice should be enabled to explore the theory and practice of clinical change, identify innovations to enhance the quality of patient care and put these into practice. Corporate recognition and support for nurse-led change and development is gradually increasing. However, top-down change is still frequently imposed with little value or due regard for the wisdom of practitioners or without an in-depth understanding of the complexity of change in dynamic clinical settings.

Change can be difficult and complex, and to be successful in practice it needs to be clearly understood. One approach to undertaking nurse-led change and development is proposed: the use of the exploratory, creative, innovative and empowering process of action research. The use of the approach should demonstrate the underlying values, concerns and clinical practice commitments of nurses. The research process - of reflecting in and on practice, identifying patient-focused issues, devising an action plan, implementing the action plan and evaluating its effectiveness - shares much in common with frameworks for clinical nursing practice, particularly the nursing process. The need therefore to adopt an action research methodology is almost self-evident. As a result, practitioners should also be better equipped to cope with the implementation of national and local policy initiatives, which include shared clinical governance and evidence-based nursing practice, both of which are evident in this text. The use of an action research approach is also recommended for advanced/higher-level

---

*A number of terms are now used for 'patient', for example 'user', 'client', 'consumer' and 'participant in care'. I have chosen to remain with 'patient', the focus being the person rather than the label.

nurse practitioners (Manley and Bellman 2000) as they are expected to lead the utilisation of research findings and implementation of evidence-based practice by nursing colleagues (Woods 2000).

Undertaking nurse-led change and development came from my desire to research patient-focused issues with my colleagues in clinical practice, and this book has been adapted from the original study (Bellman 1999). There are many approaches to change and interpretations of action research. I hoped that the systematic implementation of the critical action research approach would not only benefit patients and practitioners but also enhance team working, and multi-professional collaboration, and that the process and outcomes would ultimately be recognised and valued within the organisation. The text demonstrates the personal development process for both practitioners (called co-researchers) and the action research facilitator (myself) resulting from engaging in collaborative change in clinical practice. Also identified are the many disempowering processes (both actual and imagined) that currently exist in healthcare settings.

Two hospitals were used for the study. The settings were a surgical ward and a day surgery unit (DSU). However, the principles and practice of critical action research can be applied to all healthcare settings. In the first hospital I was an 'insider action researcher', as I was known to the directorate/unit staff in my role as lecturer in nursing. In the second hospital I was an 'outsider', with no prior knowledge of the organisation, the setting or the staff. The two interesting, important and challenging roles are explored and compared. A framework to advance nurse-led change and development in clinical practice evolved from the study.

Approaching the text

There is no standard approach to writing up an action research study. Each study should demonstrate the reality of working, learning and researching together, and 'should succeed in bringing the situation to life but (at the same time) bring out its aims and emergent general themes - methodological, professional, personal, developmental' (Clarke et al. 1993, 490).

The first two chapters consider knowledge required for undertaking nurse-led change and development. Chapter 1 explores the context for change and action research within healthcare organisations. The organisational culture, the complexities of empowerment and the extent to which nurses feel and are able to be empowered in their workplace are examined as well as the growing interest in action research in healthcare. Chapter 2 explores literature on change, action research, collaboration and facilitation. Different action research approaches are considered, particularly the usefulness of critical action research to systematically explore collaborative change and development in practice.

The Roper, Logan and Tierney model for nursing is the focus for the first study in the surgical directorate. Chapter 3 explores the potential integration of theory and practice through the controversial literature on nursing models. Preparation for the first study, in chapter 4, includes the difficulties of obtaining permission to conduct the study, the development and implementation of exploratory research tools regarding the model of nursing, presentation of the findings to the directorate nursing staff and selection of the co-researchers. Chapters 5 and 6 present a comprehensive account of the critical action research process. This includes reflecting on the model to identify patient-focused innovation, exploring the evidence for change, planning, implementing and evaluating the changes, and identifying the outcomes for the patients, nurses (co-researchers), the nurse manager, action researcher, clinical area and the hospital.

Chapters 7, 8 and 9 describe the second study in the DSU. Chapter 7 consolidates knowledge from the first study before describing how the second study originated and was then set up. The focus of the second study, the need for a dedicated day for paediatric care, is explored in chapter 8 through searching the evidence in the literature and developing a questionnaire for all the staff of the unit. Chapter 9 explores the analysis of the questionnaire and the feedback meeting with the staff. In chapter 10 the two studies are compared. Power issues are identified as well as the significant outcomes for the co-researchers and the managers. A framework for nurse-led change and development is presented from the analysis of all the process and outcome data of the two studies and from supporting literature.

The final chapter represents my personal reflections as both an insider and outsider research facilitator. It also provides guidance for critical action researchers in clinical settings. Future perspectives reflect the extent to which all practitioners will be enabled to participate in nurse-led change and development for both continuous quality improvement and professional advancement.

Chapter 1
The context for nurse-led change and development

'Nurses are responsible for the majority of the professional healthcare provided in the UK ... however, they continue to be invisible in health policy debates in both political and academic fora, because of their powerlessness.' (Maslin-Prothero and Masterson 1998)

Introduction

Nurse-led research in practice that results in change and development should be understood and valued for many reasons. It is patient-focused, collaborative, contributes to personal development and advances professional practice knowledge. In a politically driven healthcare system, it also contributes to the clinical governance agenda through continuous professional development and the identification, planning, implementation and evaluation of quality initiatives. Although nurse-led change and development can often be very challenging, it is also highly rewarding. Its importance should not be underestimated. Every day, nurses identify patient-focused problems that need addressing, and they provide common-sense resolutions that should be investigated. For example

E-grade staff nurse: *I have just had a child I could not control* [in the day surgery unit] *and I am not paediatric trained. He was a nightmare that child, hit everybody. I couldn't do a thing with him. I also had another child who I was told could go 'flat' ... Three others were grizzling. I was at the point where I wanted to go in the corner and grizzle myself. We have two paediatric-*

1

trained nurses, but neither was on duty. If we had a
dedicated day for paediatrics, they could be the leaders
of the team that day.
G-grade ward manager: *I threw two lots of her pills*
away that day. She got me so confused I wasn't sure I'd
given her the right ones. I feel anxiety [about her
impending major surgery] *was making her behave like*
that. She resented giving us her pills on admission,
complains that we never give them to her at the right
time. Well, now we just show her every bottle. I suppose
it would be better for her to do it herself but we're not
allowed to do it. Well, there is self-medication, but I
don't think pharmacy would allow us.

This book, adapted from a thesis (Bellman 1999), demonstrates the process and outcomes of nurse-led research in practice in acute clinical settings in two hospitals. It explores how nurses identified patient-specific problems, challenged the status quo and systematically implemented an evidence-based change process using critical action research (Carr & Kemmis 1986). Meyer (1993a) cautions that this type of research can be problematic, and James (1993) asserts that action research models can create an impression that improving practice is simple, whereas in many instances it is complex. Indeed, there are significant practical issues, dilemmas and risks involved for both researcher/facilitator (myself) and co-researchers (nurse participants), which Oja and Smulyan (1989) refer to as 'the powerful yet messy process'. To start to address these concerns, a working knowledge of the healthcare context is required. How do healthcare organisations manage change? How relevant are the concepts of empowerment and oppression in nursing? To what extent is action research valued in healthcare?

Nurses and organisational change

Edmonstone (1995) asserts that for some twenty-five years the National Health Service (NHS) has been absorbed with how to manage change effectively. He challenges managers to adopt a different set of basic assumptions and to consider a model of change that encompasses four phases: mobilisation, empowerment, spreading the learning and embedding the change. He suggests that humility is needed to abandon inflexible solutions and that managers need to let an overall strategy emerge, wherever possible, from successful action, building from the ground up and being opportunistic and incremental with a strong focus on action, experimentation and innovation - with regular breaks for review (looking back to see what has been learned) and planning (what to do next) (Edmonstone 1995, 19).

This proposed model for change reflects the critical action research process (Bellman 2001). Yet how realistic is this approach in health-care settings? It may take some considerable time for many healthcare managers to adopt a different set of assumptions and working practices given their style of leadership and the variety of influences that impinge on their decision-making ability.

An increasing number of approaches to change are advocated within the healthcare literature, but these broad models of change management continue to be recycled with very few new insights. Quantitative studies have dominated research on change manage-ment. Yet many of the most useful studies are well-conducted qualita-tive studies (Iles and Sutherland 2001). These authors also differentiate between the nature of evidence in the field of change management and that which is relevant and useful in the clinical arena. In this book nurse-led change and development encompasses Lewin's approach, which continues to be a popular framework for both macro and micro change situations (Wright 1996; Iles 1997), and action research, which is clearly relevant for change and improvement in healthcare organisations:

> Perhaps the most successful strategies for change may be those which focus at the level of the system, and aim to change group or team behaviours and practices by tackling specific, known problems and using a consis-tent and well-grounded methodology to do so. (Walshe 2000, 171)

In the United Kingdom there has been a growing awareness that bottom-up approaches should be advanced. Government validation of this approach is evident:

> To succeed in the NHS of the future, NHS Trusts [hospi-tals] will need to develop and involve their staff. In the past this has not been a high priority. In the new NHS it is - for one simple reason. The health service relies on the commitment and motivation of its staff. That is why

> there will be a new approach to better valuing of staff,
> and NHS Trusts will spearhead it. (Department of Health
> 1997, 50)

Yet what evidence is there to demonstrate this change in organisational culture?

Often nurses have viewed change as threatening, especially when they have not been involved in the decision to change, when they have felt undervalued in their work or have perceived change to be a criticism of their past practices (Towell and Harries 1979). Several authors, including Iles (1997), liken painful experiences of change to that of the Kubler-Ross (1969) model of loss and bereavement. Concepts include denial, anger, grief, resignation and acceptance. Cavanagh (1996) asserts that, while there appears to be little empirical evidence for this analogy, it is likely that individuals who fail to accept the reality of change will exhibit unproductive behaviour. He proposes that individual responses to change can be considered on a continuum from broadly positive support through to deliberate sabotage.

Within the literature on changing practice, Pryjmachuk (1996) encourages not only the analysis of positive processes and outcomes of an action research study but also the analysis of failures. This approach was used by Allen (1996), in his role as a nursing-process training officer, to identify how change could have been handled more sensitively and successfully. The effects of the mismanagement of change are still felt and observed by him many years later.

In their action research study to facilitate institutional change, East and Robinson (1994) found that the nurses were motivated to change. Yet hospital managers' and senior ward nurses' differing perceptions, financial constraints and crisis management defied all attempts at continuity of care and changing practice. The authors concluded that nurses should not underestimate the pain that is involved when exploring change. It requires the researchers/facilitators to make the political issues of power and control explicit and to explore to the limits the common ground that exists.

The above are just a few of many examples that demonstrate the need to understand the complexities of the change process and, in particular, the extent to which nurses feel able to, and are empowered to, undertake nurse-led change and development in healthcare organisations.

Empowerment and oppression in nursing

The concepts of empowerment and oppression have increasingly featured in nursing literature. These concepts are linked to complex historical, political, social, cultural and economic forces that currently exist within nursing. The need for nurse empowerment has resulted from the 'political climate of oppression' (Farmer 1993), which has created a tension between the values of a financial market philosophy and the care and concern for humanity. Issues of oppression and empowerment have been linked with nurse leaders, healthcare managers, the medical profession and nurse educators. There is also a need to explore the conceptual ambiguity of empowerment (Gilbert 1995). Indeed, NHS reports state that the Government will empower local doctors, nurses and health authorities to meet the needs of local patients (Department of Health 1997) and will empower frontline staff to develop innovative services to meet those needs (Department of Health 2001). Yet there is no agreement on the meaning of empowerment.

Fulton (1997) explores how empowerment was understood by sixteen nurses. This process complemented a unit of learning that was designed to 'meet the challenge of developing an empowered and empowering practitioner'. This approach was seen as a bold and radical innovation within a curriculum based on critical social theories. The thematic content analysis from the sixteen nurses (who made up two separate focus groups) revealed the following categories: empowerment related to decision-making, choice, authority; having personal power related to assertiveness, knowledge and experience; relationships within the multidisciplinary team reflecting medical power, limited autonomy; feeling right about oneself, reflecting confidence, low self-esteem and being manipulative. Overall, Fulton (1997) found that the nurses in her study saw empowerment in terms of freedom - the freedom to make decisions with authority and to have choices.

The previous year Rodwell (1996) published a concept analysis of empowerment which was drawn from a multifaceted literature that encompassed nursing, education, management, environment, sociology, psychology and feminism. The attributes of empowerment that she identifies (table 1.1) are similar to Fulton's (1997) findings, but the extent to which nurses are able to implement them remains controversial.

Table 1.1: The attributes of empowerment (Rodwell 1996).

- a helping process
- a partnership that values self and others
- mutual decision-making, using resources, opportunities and authority
- freedom to make choices and accept responsibility

Indeed, in practice, empowerment is more easily understood by its absence, which is characterised by powerlessness, helplessness, alienation, victimisation, subordination and oppression (Gibson 1991). To focus on nurses as oppressed, as victims, has the potential to devalue a professional group whose strength is predominantly the holistic care of the individual. Yet there is evidence within the literature to support the oppression of nurses by powerful groups, the most significant of whom appear to be have been nurse leaders.

Nurse leaders

Quinn (1989) believes that nursing leaders should be convinced of the need to work with the grassroots, allowing the initiatives to come from the periphery. Yet, historically, nursing has 'developed a system of oppressing its own because the nursing hierarchy couldn't cope with anything that was outside of command and control' (Asbridge 2001, 18). Farmer (1993), in her exploration of the use and abuse of power in nursing, is primarily concerned by the hard core of nurse leaders whose thirst for power and personal ambition often cause them to act at the expense of the common good.

> We have to find a way to help the 'queen bees' [and male equivalents] in our discipline to recognise that power comes only through the empowerment of others. (Farmer 1993, 36)

Previous condemnation of nurse leaders (Roberts 1983) exemplified them as an elite and marginal group who were promoted because of their allegiance to maintaining the status quo. A more recent view on empowerment for nurses (Hamilton-Hurren 1997) raises similar concerns. Some nurse leaders are berated for their lack of recognition of nursing values and systems of care, as well as their lack of cohesive identity, mutual trust and support.

Roberts (1983) challenges nurse leaders to recognise the existence of oppression and to motivate nurses to imagine the unimagined and become aware of their social conditioning. In some instances the opposite appears to have occurred. O'Kelly (1994) and Bowman (1997) are highly critical of those nurse leaders who have isolated themselves, who over-manage nurses rather than lead and manage nursing, and who underestimate the value of the job nurses do. The consequence has been to disempower nursing. Nurse leaders appear to have aligned themselves with the more powerful groups, i.e. medicine and the management hierarchy. Yet, no matter how much the nurse manager identifies with the empowered group, nurses will still find that they have the least amount of power among them (O'Kelly 1994). Nurse leaders need to identify, develop and implement empowering processes that reflect nursing values at all levels of the organisation.

Successful empowerment depends upon excellent leadership (Hamilton-Hurren 1997), but nurse leaders are also portrayed as disenfranchised and vulnerable (Andrews-Evans 1997). Strategies for the liberation of nursing executives are advocated by Roberts (1997). Her advice is intended to reverse the cycle of low self-esteem and internalised hostility that has led, as she sees it, to much of the negativity and divisiveness in nursing. Nurses are not to be viewed as inherently inferior, yet they have been placed in a culture that devalues their attributes. This awareness should not be a depressing one but rather a call to action based on the development of a shared set of values and goals.

Yet liberating leaders should not force empowerment onto unwilling shoulders; 'they [should] create the environment in which both the timid and the bold can take more responsibility and accountability for their actions knowing that they will not be abandoned in times of strain or trouble' (Tampoe 1998, 4). This new way of working could resemble a multidimensional approach to leadership (Bate 1994, table 1.2).

The multidimensional approach demonstrates the need for empowering processes even though it does not explicitly address the antecedents of empowerment, which Rodwell (1996) identifies as mutual trust and respect, education and support, and participation and

---

Table 1.2: A multidimensional leadership approach (adapted from Bate 1994).

The dimensions of the 'new' leadership

1.	**Aesthetic**	The leader *assists* in the creation, expression and communication of a new idea or explication of a problem.
2.	**Political**	The leader *assists* in inscribing those ideas into a body of socially agreed meanings and engages in empowering processes.
3.	**Ethical**	The leader *assists* in developing and imparting to others a framework of moral standards governing the expression and development of these meanings and ideas.
4.	**Action**	The leader *assists* in the process of transmuting the agreed cultural meanings into concrete cultural practices.
5.	**Formative**	The leader *assists* in structuring these meanings and collaborative practices into some kind of rationale or framework.

commitment. These antecedents are fundamental within the critical action research approach. A leader who 'assists' others (table 1.2) demonstrates an empowering, less directive approach. Indeed, empowerment within a multidimensional leadership approach can be viewed as returning power and control to practitioners, which McConnell (1995) refers to as 'delegation done well'. The approach should also enhance the interpersonal process element of empowerment, which Rodwell (1996) believes practitioners appear to value. However, if nurse leaders are to adopt this type of approach, they also need the recognition and support of senior healthcare/corporate managers and administrators.

Managers

Different interest groups within healthcare organisations may place different meanings on the same term. Hence, *empowerment* in managerial terms is seen as a means towards managerial ends rather than (from a professional perspective) a desirable end in itself (Edmonstone 2000). Waite (1997) highlights the continued lack of recognition for nurses by top-level NHS administrators, which contributes to low morale. This lack of recognition and support has been, according to Caine and Kenrick (1997), a recognised strategy to empower managers at the expense of professionals:

> General managers were almost evangelical in their desire to change what they described as the traditional culture among nurses and other professional groups by breaking down professional boundaries, and yet paradoxically were protective of their own professional territory and status. (Hart and Bond 1995, 108)

More recent literature demonstrates an oppressive culture:

> I expected to find this group of empowered nurses who were very much a team, who had decided that this was what they wanted and were very much into developing practice, but, of course, I didn't find anything like that. What I did find ... was a group of demoralised, unmotivated, powerless individuals ... The managerial structures within the [GP] practice and the [NHS] Trust were disempowering. There was a very tight, very close form of governance. Everything had to be checked before a decision was made about anything. (Burke 1998, 14)

Even so, Government reports (Department of Health 1997, 1999) refer to greater involvement of staff, strengthening of the nursing contribution and the need for open communication and collaboration. A recommendation from the *Principles into Practice Report* (British Association of Medical Managers 1996), endorsed by the British Medical Association, Institute of Health Services Management and the Royal College of Nursing and supported by the NHS Executive, states that a fundamentally healthy organisation involves its staff in the day-to-day operations and decisions that affect them and is effective and responsive. Also:

> There is a need to draw on the wisdom and experience of clinical staff and practitioners; in particular, they need to be encouraged to look at ways of improving the cost or quality of what they do, and they may need help and support in developing new approaches. In the end, only practitioners are able to come up with genuine options for change. (British Association of Medical Managers 1996, 48)

The recognition to support the majority of nurses rather than the few is in contrast to previous Government initiatives. In the 1980s thirty nursing development units (NDUs) were established by the Department of Health. The aim of these pioneering units was to encourage innovation through excellence in practice. The nurses within the units pursued and, in many instances, achieved this aim. However, the well-respected, nationally recognised NDU in Oxford was eventually disbanded through management and medical intervention.

The Scope of Professional Practice, to enable nurses to determine their own professional boundaries, was launched by the UKCC in 1992. The launch coincided with the Government's awareness of the need to reduce junior doctors' hours. As a result, and increasingly, the new specialist roles that nurses adopted - for example as nurse anaesthetists (Audit Commission 1997), surgeons' assistants (Tuthill 1995), nurse endoscopists (UKCC 1997) - appeared to support the needs of management and medicine rather than nurse/patient-focused development (Dimond 1995). In the community, and as a direct result of the white papers 'Promoting Better Health' (Department of Social Security 1987) and 'Working for Patients' (Department of Health 1989) and the *GP Contract* (Health Education Authority 1990), the focus on health promotion enabled the recognition of practice nurses (United Kingdom Central Council 1990). The nurse practitioner role evolved because of the projected shortfall in the number of general practitioners. The past two decades of national and local role development in nursing, including the development of the consultant nurse (Manley 1997), appear to have advanced professional knowledge, enabled personal and professional empowerment and, most importantly, have the potential to enhance the quality of service provision. Nevertheless, these initiatives, in the main, still only reflect the professional development of a minority of nurses.

Medical staff

If nurses are to feel and be empowered to participate in change, they will need to value their contribution and to feel valued as partners in care with medical staff. Yet the nurses in Fulton's (1997) study felt that their autonomy was seriously limited by unequal power relationships with medical staff. There is an international body of literature that addresses perceived and actual inequality in professional status and practice between nurses and doctors. Street (1995, 14) found that a closer examination of the power relationships in clinical and research activities demonstrated that medical dominance was alive and well. Historians such as Porter (1997, 647) have explored the power and influence of the medical profession with 'hospitals as the great power-base for the medical elite'. Meyer (1995) in her action research study states that she wanted to take a multidisciplinary approach to innovating change on the ward but even at the early stage of the action research project, hierarchical barriers between doctors and nurses were encountered.

Most of Fulton's (1997, 532-533) research revealed issues with doctors, for example: 'The nurses seemed to believe that they needed rational knowledge such as doctors have in order to be empowered. Doctors were seen as unapproachable and difficult to correct.'

Nurses often describe medical domination but do not attempt to analyse why it occurs. An understanding of historical and political forces is required. For example, Porter's (1997) account of medical history regarding maternal and child mortality in the early twentieth century reveals physicians' gut prejudices and professional esprit de corps - for, rather than initiate the safer home delivery practices of midwives, they chose to believe that hospitals provided the best that science could offer.

> How could mere midwives provide safer deliveries than top physicians? - midwives ... were filthy and ignorant and not far removed from the jungles. (Porter 1997, 712)

Freidson (1988) explores the differences and similarities between medicine and paramedical occupations. He concludes that it is the physician's control of the division of labour that is distinct. In nursing, it was Florence Nightingale who recognised nursing as a formal part of the doctor's work. Nursing was thus defined as a subordinate part of the technical division of labour surrounding medicine. The challenge since has been to attempt to increase nursing's power-base within the field of healthcare. New nursing roles may go some way towards empowering nurses. A more hopeful perspective has been provided by three doctors. They revisited the political and social changes that surround the 'doctor-nurse game'. The doctors conclude:

> Physicians and nurses can both benefit if their relation-
> ship becomes more mutually interdependent.
> Subservient and dominant roles are both psychologically
> restricting. When a subordinate becomes liberated,
> there is potential for the dominant one to become liber-
> ated too. (Stein et al. 1990, 549)

There is international confirmation regarding nurses feeling under-valued and disempowered by medical staff. In North America, Coeling and Wilcox (1994) report on a survey of 1,100 nurses. Over half of the nurses reported that they did not think that physicians understood nursing; the nurses felt that they were in a subordinate role to them rather than in a collegial partnership. Adamson et al. (1995) developed and administered a nurses' self-perception scale to 108 British and 133 Australian nurses. The scale was based on an exhaustive review of nursing literature and consisted of a sixty-nine-item questionnaire covering aspects of doctor-nurse, doctor-patient, nurse-patient and nurse-hospital administrative relationships. Internal consistency of the different items on the scale was evidenced by a Cronbach alpha range of 0.91-0.72.

While acknowledging that Australian nurses felt somewhat less disempowered than their British counterparts, the findings revealed that overall the nurses felt that they lacked control over allocation of funds, and they were not considered as professional equals by doctors or other healthcare professionals who did not understand nurses' work. They also did not feel respected by hospital administrators or the medical profession. They perceived the medical profession to have more political influence and more control over funding and patient management. In conclusion, it was medical dominance in both countries that was perceived to be a barrier to workplace satisfaction.

There are signs of change. An empowering initiative by a hospital enabled nurses to be involved in the planning and delivery of a course in day surgery for medical students. According to Seabrook (1998), they were motivated by the belief that their teaching would help to break down barriers between doctors and nurses. Previous positive outcomes of learning from nurses had been reported by Casey and Smith (1997) in the *British Medical Journal*, and interprofessional learning is increasingly seen as a way of sharing knowledge and promoting understanding between different professional groups.

Another important and potentially empowering process for nurses, the advancement of the patient advocacy role, is explored by Sines (1994). He notes the challenges by doctors against nurse advocacy, as they presume that it is their responsibility to discuss issues relating to diagnosis and prognosis. Nurses are seen as inadequately prepared for the responsibilities of advocacy. He believes that relegating the nursing role to subservient status preserves the 'power-base' of the medical profession. The issue is complex. Sills (1993) describes how as a patient's advocate she challenged a consultant's decision to use a lotion (which research evidence had demonstrated could contribute to tissue damage):

> We sought professional advice from the Royal College of Nursing who strongly supported our stand, but the United Kingdom Central Council stated that we were on difficult ground. As the consultant had prescribed the treatment we would be in breach of our code not to carry it out ... I felt the consultant was not ready to listen to the nurses' view. This only fuelled my determination to prove that as nurses we had a say in the patient's treatment and that we would advocate the rights of our patient because the patient himself was unable to do so ... We received little support in the hospital ... We had no alternative but to use the lotion. (Sills 1993, 4)

The example above demonstrates that, while in most organisations power is unequally shared between stakeholders, within healthcare organisations the unequal balance of power between the medical profession and other healthcare workers is ubiquitous (Johnson and Scholes 1993) and all too often a major barrier to change (Minor 1998). A literature review on nurse-doctor relationships (Sweet and Norman 1995) identifies and reinforces the traditional patriarchal pattern. Conversely, an earlier report in a medical journal reveals that, although, at one time, the relationship was hierarchic, doctors were dominant and in charge - nurses were their handmaidens; they were subordinate, subservient and often submissive - now things were starting to change:

> The new doctor-nurse relationship is characterised by the co-existence of self-directed professionals who are complementary and independent but also autonomous.
> (Smith, 1990, 218)

The recognition for change is commendable, but strategies for change are virtually nonexistent. Sweet and Norman (1995) provide no constructive practical advice from their literature review regarding the future. Minor (1998) berates nurses for adopting a passive, nonassertive role and hence propagating power and control by doctors. Meanwhile, Warelow (1997) believes this 'culture of silence' is understandable. For many nurses, to confront the patriarchal system (and bureaucracy) may prove too difficult at the moment. He believes that a knowledge of critical theory and self-reflection will enable nurses to recognise the domination, repression and ideological constraints on their thoughts and actions. M.C. Smith (1990) advances a stage further by suggesting that healthcare professionals should reflect on their practice together and, if necessary, change what they do and how they do it. Both approaches should be adopted and underpin the critical action research approach. This should enable the outcomes of empowerment (table 1.3) to be realised. There is increasing evidence that research into achieving these outcomes is urgently required. Lumby (1996) describes the daily exodus of bedside nurses who are 'voting with their feet by leaving nursing for alternative employment where they feel valued'.

Table 1.3: The outcomes of empowerment (Rodwell 1996).

Positive self-esteem
Sense of hope for the future
The ability to set and reach goals
Have a sense of control over life and the change processes

Educators

At a local level there is agreement that nurse educators could expose the oppressive structures which confine and limit the nursing experience (Harden 1996, Fulton 1997). A key strategy is to promote an environment where nurses can communicate freely, but this is perceived as a revolutionary approach in hospitals, which are considered 'the bastions of patriarchal bureaucracy and control, with [their] hierarchical communication systems' (Harden 1996).

Duffy and Scott (1998) identify the need for collaborative reflection by education and clinical staff to explore their unequal power relationship. They also wish to explore other oppressive structures within both education and practice. The nature of empowerment within this approach is about enabling nurses to realise and use their own power to effect change. Many nurses appear to be uncomfortable with the idea of power (Warelow 1996). Yet Conway (1996), in the foreword to her book, asserts:

> If the selective blindness of the oppressed is to be overcome nurses need to be empowered so that they can cope with looking searchingly at themselves and their practice. Empowerment is much more than a popular cliché of the moment.

This approach is clearly evident within the action research study undertaken by Street (1995), a sociologist and educator. She enabled nurses to challenge the control myths that are sustained through language practices, moral judgements and value stances, which are also often unexpressed and unacknowledged. Disempowering habitual language patterns were identified (Street 1995, 18-19), for example: 'No, he is not a doctor. He is *just* a nurse!' and 'I hate hurting children but they *have* to have these painful procedures, and I *can't* change anything.' This last example reflects both disempowerment and an ethical dilemma for the nurse.

Oppressed group?

The literature demonstrates that nurses are often portrayed as an oppressed group. Educators have begun to identify the need to explore empowering strategies. On top of this, it is essential that all nurses understand how managers, doctors and nurses themselves have contributed to their disempowerment and oppression. The view shared by many authors, including Warelow (1996), is that nurses are socially conditioned to accept taken-for-granted cultural norms - institutional rules and routines which enable them to participate willingly in their own domination, often without even recognising it. Street (1995) recommends listening to one's own comments and examining values in action as important ways of uncovering practices that are entrenched in culturally created habitual attitudes and disempowering language.

Nursing values may often be suppressed by political forces, managerial issues and medical tasks. For some nurse leaders, their nursing values may appear to have been discarded. Meyer (1995) warns that changing practice raises the sensitive issue of people with vested interests maintaining the status quo. To enable nurse-led change and development, nursing values need to be rediscovered, shared and employed at all levels of the organisation.

Nurses may believe they have little power within the organisation; yet they wield considerable power when caring for patients. Thus, empowerment is a complex concept that can be analysed from many differing perspectives.

The complexities of empowerment

Within the social work literature, Parsloe (1997) considers the ethical issues related to the exercise of social power. She states that the principle of empowerment is central to the exercise of social power but, equally, is qualified by the limitations of all those involved and the pre-existing situation. 'There is no right answer but equally there is no neutral position' (Parsloe 1997, 10). Currently nurses are perceived to exert a great deal of power, particularly in relationships with older people, children and the mentally disabled (Suominen et al. 1997). There is enormous scope for interpreting patient empowerment, but Elliott and Turrell (1996) believe that it always involves a transfer of power from the nurse to the patient. The nurses in Fulton's (1997) study felt they could not advise, challenge or empower others until they were comfortable with themselves. Towell suggests that self-empowerment at the individual/micro level is as important as collective responsibility, which, at the macro level:

> requires not only that we share the responsibility for providing support but also that we work towards creating a society which welcomes all its members by opening up opportunities and reducing barriers to participation. (Towell 1996, 296)

The issue is highly complex, both for healthcare staff and patients. Current political legislation (Department of Health 2001) and professional organisations now recognise the need for user and staff empowerment. However, the concept and its application remain ambiguous.

An important factor in the empowerment of service users is the extent to which healthcare organisations/agencies are willing to empower their own staff (Parsloe 1997). The extent to which patient empowerment may be implemented will therefore depend on health services managers/leaders acknowledging nurses and patients in the decision-making process and in the employment of empowering strategies for nurses. The impact of perceived medical dominance is an equally significant factor. Challenging the status quo in areas where there is little recognition of empowering processes is extraordinarily difficult and may place nurses in an invidious position. Those in existing positions of authority can isolate, ignore, ridicule and make those challenging them feel guilty and unworthy (East and Robinson 1994).

Yet, as nurses continue to advance their specialist nursing roles as well as undertake the duties of a junior doctor, the message they receive is that nurses and doctors should be equal partners in planning and managing the new roles (Reports 1996). They should also be equal partners when undertaking research in practice. However, valuing applied research in clinical practice will require a significant paradigm shift.

Research paradigm shift?

The focus for nursing research reflects the current culture within NHS reforms and the research and development strategy (Department of Health 1991a) with the emphasis upon evidence-based practice. The gold standard for evidence is still the randomised control trial; although this is now being challenged (Simons 2000).

Fortunately, there is also acknowledgement of the potentially exciting use of a range of research methodologies for clinical nursing (Thompson 1998). Indeed, this view is realistic in the light of 'the messy swamp of nurses' daily activities where the most important and challenging problems arise and the ontological substance of nursing is to be found' (Retsas 1994, 24).

Hayes (1996) states that action research appears for some to be too philosophical to constitute research, as it is a creative way to obtain new insights, identify new knowledge and foster transformations of thinking. However, there is now increasing evidence within nursing and healthcare literature of the need to continue to develop knowledge of action research. The first British action research text for healthcare professionals was published in 1995 by Hart, a social anthropologist, and Bond, a social worker. They state that the current ideology of reform and improvement in the health- and social-care services, along with other related developments, points almost inevitably in the direction of action research. These current developments include growing pressure on professional staff to make use of relevant research findings, the effective deployment of scarce resources and greater accountability for actions.

According to Hart (1995), the opportunity to undertake action research seemed part of an almost natural development towards a more participatory way of working. Her training as a social anthropologist meant that initially it 'went against the grain' to intervene directly in a situation to change it. Yet intervention is seen by Johnson (1997a) as an ethical and humane approach that is required for nursing and healthcare practice research. He believes that undertaking clinical research within a positivist or interpretive paradigm is 'hygienic'. He argues that the passive collection of data from patients is in conflict with the value systems of nurses, who should facilitate changes in practice by empowering themselves and their patients. His reflections on his doctoral studies lead him to conclude:

> I am still left with a feeling that, despite the help I may
> have been able to offer, a better approach might have
> been to do the study from a more clearly action research
> perspective ... I would certainly seriously consider this
> kind of approach in the future. (Johnson 1997b)

Another advocate of action research (Pryjmachuk 1996) challenges the current purely academic analysis and debate surrounding the concept of change. He calls for a pragmatic approach to change and believes that action research is the key to effecting and understanding change/innovation. He cites the potential for effecting change in large organisations, both on a micro and macro scale:

> Nurses would do well to grasp its fundamentals, for the
> sooner that nursing embraces action research, the
> sooner we will see developments in nurses, in nursing
> practices and in the discipline of nursing as a whole.
> (Pryjmachuk 1996)

Similar views are held by Australian and New Zealand nurses. Much of their nursing literature challenges positivist science as the dominant research paradigm (FitzGerald 1995, Sutton and Smith 1995, Holmes 1996). Greenwood (1995) believes that the role of nursing research is the development and promotion of scholarship in practice through action research. The adoption of critical theory, the foundation of the critical action research approach, is advocated as a basis for education and practice. Owen-Mills (1995) refers to the transformative nurse educator who teaches caring within a critical social paradigm and has a responsibility to ensure students understand the mandate for social action. Yet

Lont (1995) concludes from her analysis of nine curricula that, while the documents largely incorporate the language of critical theory, emphasis is still on the attainment of technical/instrumental skills of old, which could be more easily taught and measured. However, she asserts that Habermasian critical social theory (see chapter 2) should be the basis for education for nurses in the twenty-first century. If the theory is to contribute to nurse education, it should logically follow that its philosophical assumptions and theoretical concepts should also guide nursing practice. In this way the theory-practice gap can be addressed.

Early advocates of the critical social theory of Habermas (chapter 2) have attempted to put into practice the philosophical approach within education action research (Grundy 1982, Carr and Kemmis 1986). Some nurses are sceptical of clinical nurses adopting other disciplines' philosophical perspectives (Huntington et al. 1996, Greenwood 1994 in Meyer and Bateup 1997). These authors advocate caution in the uncritical adoption of ideas from one discipline to another which might be appropriate for educational settings but may not be suitable for healthcare practice. Yet, Hart and Bond (1995a, 8) believe that the role of action research in nursing has parallels with that in teacher education, as both are seeking to consolidate their status as a 'profession', to develop a discrete knowledge-base for practice and to increase their control over their work in the current climate of major organisational change.

The World Health Organisation (WHO) Expert Committee's view of research appears to mirror action research approaches. They recognise that research is an activity appropriate to all levels of nursing personnel.

> To facilitate this process, opportunities should be provided for nurses at all levels of the healthcare system to examine critically the environment in which they work. At the local level, nurses can work with other healthcare providers and with communities, collecting data to identify changes in health and social needs, and to devise problem-solving strategies ... Research need not be expensive; simple, small-scale projects can be carried out by individual nurses or by small groups, even multidisciplinary ones. (WHO 1996, 20)

The WHO document also takes account of the macro socio-political context within which nursing takes place. Significant changes will need to occur within Great Britain to facilitate the WHO's collaborative research perspective. New research and development funding arrangements have provided 'windows of opportunity' for partnership developments between NHS Trusts and nursing departments within universities. Nursing Research and Development (R and D) units have been set up in some parts of the country, but these units focus, in the main, on positivist and interpretive research and are based within the confines of the university. Riley and Omery (1996) argue for the need to challenge the tradition in nursing of distinguishing between the development of knowledge in academic or research settings and its use in clinical practice. The authors' clinical scholarship approach proposes that *all* (their italics) nurses, as members of a discipline that is embedded in practice, share in the obligation to take part in the generation, utilisation and evaluation of knowledge designed to benefit the health and well-being of the people they serve. Obversely, the interpretation by Davies (1997) is that only a small proportion of each clinical profession will be active researchers.

From their exploration of action research approaches, Meyer and Bateup (1997) conclude that a paradigmatic shift is apparent even though they acknowledge that the NHS research and development strategy is being driven by a positivist understanding of science, which overemphasises outcomes and is medically driven. Yet, while the key focus of the political research agenda is evidence-based care, undertaken within a predominantly positivist methodology, current government initiatives also paradoxically advocate user involvement, patient empowerment and partnerships with patients (Department of Health 1997). These initiatives require different definitions of evidence, different research approaches and new ways of working, researching and learning.

There is certainly a growing interest in action research. A recent NHS-funded review of action research (Waterman et al. 2001) recommends that it should be considered as complementary to other research approaches within the NHS, and that it has a potential role in:

- innovation, for example in the development and evaluation of new services
- improvements in healthcare, for example monitoring the effectiveness of untested policies or interventions
- development of knowledge and understanding in practitioners and other service providers, for example promotion of informed decision-making
- involvement of users and NHS staff, for example investigations and improvement of situations in which there is poor uptake of preventative services.

Nurses are therefore well placed to do this.

Moving forward

Undertaking nurse-led change and development in clinical settings is enhanced by an understanding of the context for the integration of change, research and development in healthcare organisations. Also required is the recognition of historical factors that have contributed to the disempowerment and oppression of nurses. Many of these factors could deter nurses from changing clinical practice. However, nurses can and do enhance the quality of patient care by challenging the status quo and implementing change, preferably in a systematic way. One approach is that of critical action research, which enables nurses to recognise and value their own self-worth, to understand the forces that impinge on their expertise, professional judgement and development, and to acquire the appropriate knowledge and skills to effect change in their clinical setting.

Chapter 2
Evolving clinical change and action research

'Managing change is crucial to the survival of every staff
nurse, manager, teacher and administrator in healthcare
today.' (Lancaster 1999)

Fundamentals of change

A knowledge of the theory and practice of change can enhance nurse-led change and development in practice. Central to the process of change, but rarely discussed, are the concerns of power, influence, politics and conflict (Cope 1981). These issues, which are briefly explored in chapter 1, must be addressed to enable nurses to be proactive, influence decision-making and empower themselves and their patients. A knowledge of change theories, critical social theory and action research can begin to address these issues. The approach to practitioner research is complex because of the many interacting people, factors and forces involved (Lancaster 1999). Tiffany and Lutjens caution:

> Change is difficult ... Change is inevitable. We ignore
> change at our peril ... Careful planning increases the
> probability of fruitful outcomes and decreases the likeli-
> hood of disaster. Careful planning requires thoughtful
> study. (1998, 3)

The origin of classical change theory is attributed to Kurt Lewin (Tiffany and Lutjens 1998). Three steps are described in the change process - unfreezing, moving, refreezing. *Unfreezing* is motivating participants in the direction of readiness for change by 'thawing them out'. During this phase, participants recognise the need for a change,

21

work to diagnose the problem and generate a solution by selecting from a number of alternative approaches. The second phase, *moving*, involves changing and developing new beliefs, values and attitudes on the basis of new information and insights. Cognitive redefinition occurs due to collecting sufficient information about the situation (evidence for change) and recognising the need to alter the status quo and agreeing on an action plan. *Refreezing* occurs when the newly acquired behaviour is integrated into the participants' personalities (Lancaster 1999). During this stage, positive feedback, encouragement and constructive criticism reinforce newly learned behaviour (Olsen 1979).

Lewin's theory is expanded upon by Rogers (1962). Rogers emphasises both the background of people participating in the change process and the environment in which the change takes place. Lewin's concepts of driving and restraining forces (see table 2.1) also evolved and have been usefully employed in many change strategies.

From the wealth of literature addressing strategies for change, many authors believe that a particularly significant factor is to determine the perceived need for change (Cope 1981, Wright 1998). Unfortunately, when change strategies have been implemented in hospitals, the staff's and users' perspectives have not always been key influencing factors.

Table 2.1: Lewin's Force Field Analysis categories.

FORCE FIELD ANALYSIS

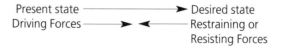

Present state ——————————➤ Desired state
Driving Forces ——————➤ ◄—————— Restraining or
Resisting Forces

Categories of Forces

Technological
Economic
Political
Socio-cultural

Organisational
Policy
Structural

Group
Interpersonal

Individual/Person

From their planned change in hospital studies, Bennis et al. (1985) identify three deliberate change strategies and their theoretical bases - rational-empirical, normative-re-educative and power-coercive (see table 2.2).

While it would appear that the normative-re-educative strategy would be most appropriate for changing nursing practice, Swan and McVicar (1992) caution against following a single model or one strategy, because it may well be inhibiting. They recognise that there is always great effort invested in the content of any proposed change; yet the *process* of change is rarely taken into account or explored.

The complex process of change should be part of the knowledge-base of all nurses, educators and managers. A key part of the strategy for exploring change and development, particularly within action research approaches, is reflective practice.

Table 2.2: Approaches to change and their theoretical bases (adapted from Wright 1989).

Change strategies	Beliefs	Common assumption	Approaches
Rational-empirical	All persons are guided by reason.	The belief that the dissemination of research findings will change nursing practice.	Top-down
Power-coercive	Knowledge is a major source and ingredient of power.	People with less power will always comply with the plans, directives and leadership of those with more power.	Top-down
Normative-re-educative	People need to be involved in all aspects of the change process; their actions are directed by a normative culture.	Changes in practice involve the individual's or group's perceptions of the need for change and its relationship to daily practices.	Bottom-up

Reflective practice

Boud et al. (1985) state that reflection comprises those intellectual and affective activities in which individuals engage in order to explore their experiences to reach new understandings and appreciations. Reflective practice involves practitioners who can draw from a range of theories in a creative way, to address the particular, unique and complex problems that they face in practice (Reed and Procter 1993). Reflective practice would therefore imply that not only is a self-critique important but a critique of the institutional context is also required. Kemmis (1985) believes that reflection is not a purely creative exercise but a practice which expresses our power to reconstitute social life by the way we participate in communication, decision-making and social action. Reflection is seen to serve human interest and therefore in this sense is political. Habermas (1972) shows that this search for knowledge is guided by different kinds of self-interest. The three broad types of interest (associated with each of the Aristolian forms of reason), are technical, practical and emancipatory. Their classification and characteristics are summarised in table 2.3. These three forms of human interest underpin the positivist/empirical-analytical, interpretive phenomenological and critical social theory research methodologies.

Table 2.3: Classification and characteristics of human interests (adapted from Kemmis 1985).

Interest	Knowledge	Medium of social organisation	Science	Actions
Technical	Instrumental: causal explanation	Work	Empirical-analytic (physical sciences)	Problem-solving
Practical	Practical: understanding	Language	Hermeneutic or interpretive science (history)	Wise action in a social context
Emancipatory	Critical: critique	Power	Critical social science	Social action towards emancipation

Schon (1983) uses the term *technical rationality* to label theoretical knowledge developed in an academic setting that has been separated from practice. Reed and Procter (1993) suggest that Schon's description is extremely relevant to past and current debates about the knowledge-base of nursing. In 1975 Schlotfeldt criticised nursing knowledge as being at an intuitive level. Three years later, Carper identified ethical, aesthetic, empirical and personal ways of knowing. More recently, Benner (1984) has advocated a return to the more abstract, tacit and personal areas of knowledge. Reflection therefore could enable nurses to extrapolate different ways of knowing in practice, and become familiar with the rules and traditions of oppression (Maggs-Rapport 2001) (see chapter 1). While this is worthwhile on an individual basis, within an action research approach, 'collaborative discourse and shared reflections are often far more productive and potentially liberating than isolated introspection' (Cox et al. 1991, 385).

Johns (1993) demonstrates how reflective practice could promote creative, effective, therapeutic work with patients. He utilises a case-study approach and adopts the role of clinical facilitator to primary nurses. Yet he concludes by identifying five barriers to achieving effect-iveness, which may still be considered relevant in some healthcare settings:

1. Hierarchical-bureaucratic organisational systems in nursing that emphasise conformity to role and status and limit opportunity for responsibility and creativity.
2. Existing social systems to protect nurses from anxiety that have fostered an avoidance of decision-making, sharing feelings, taking responsibility and therapeutic relationships with patients.
3. The manner of nurse education that has conditioned nurses to feel subordinate and powerless.
4. The situation of women in society where the dominant values are seen as masculine and caring is viewed as an extension of domestic work with low social value - leading to low self-esteem and passivity.
5. The relationship to medicine that has limited nursing's ability to define and fulfil its therapeutic role and hence has led to nursing viewing itself as subordinate and powerless to change.

A similar situation in North America (Rogers 1989) refers to nurses undervaluing their knowledge and skills, their capacity to effect change and the continued use of the medical model as their conceptual model for practice. Smyth (1987) believes that most people are unlikely to change and usually adopt the line of least resistance. Yet Cox et al. (1991) assert that, as it exposes the forces which dominate and constrain nursing from realising its potential, critical reflection exposes new ways of knowing and new ways of acting within that world. However, the authors do acknowledge that engaging in critical reflection takes courage and a willingness to step into the uncomfortable world of the, as yet, unknown.

For reflective practice to lead to new understandings and actions an emancipatory approach (table 2.3) should be adopted to facilitate the process. Eby (2000) asserts that reflective practice entails the synthesis of self-awareness, reflection and critical thinking. Critical practitioners, according to Brechin (2000), must be skilled and knowledgeable and yet remain open to alternative ideas, frameworks and belief systems, recognising and valuing alternative perspectives. These views are fundamental to engaging in collaborative nurse-led change and development within an emancipatory or critical action research approach.

The advancement of action research

Kurt Lewin, as well as being the originator of classical change theory, also first coined the phrase 'action research' in the mid-1940s as a result of participating in community projects in post-war America and studying broader social issues. However, there are now a number of different approaches; consequently, action research is not easily defined (Meyer and Bateup 1997) and there is little agreement about what it means. It is interesting to note that in 1990 the *Dictionary of Nursing Theory and Research* (Powers and Knapp 1990) had no entries under the letter A. The second edition includes 'action research' and 'applied research'. Powers (1995, 1) succinctly defines action research as:

> Applied research that is oriented towards producing
> innovation and change. It can be self-evaluative and
> autobiographical, involving, for example, examination
> of one's own caring practices or teaching activities; or it
> can be collective, emphasising the role of participants as
> partners and stakeholders in studies that are responsive
> to their interests and concerns.

This definition, while understating the 'democratic, equitable, liberating and life enhancing' characteristics of action research (Stringer 1996, 10), clearly differentiates between the individual and collaborative approaches.

A systematic review of action research (Waterman et al. 2001) has led to a lengthier definition (box 2.1).

The action research process begins with a general idea that some kind of change is desirable. McTaggart (1982, 7) describes the four 'moments' or fundamental aspects of the process:

Box 2.1: Definition of action research (Waterman et al. 2001).

Action research is a period of inquiry that describes, interprets and explains social situations while executing a change intervention aimed at improvement and involvement. It is problem-focused, context-specific and future-orientated. Action research is a group activity with an explicit critical value basis and is founded on a partnership between action researchers and participants, all of whom are involved in the change process. The participatory process is educative and empowering, involving a dynamic approach in which problem identification, planning, action and evaluation are inter-linked. Knowledge may be advanced through reflection and research, and qualitative and quantitative research methods may be employed to collect data. Different types of knowledge, including practical and prepositional [theories, facts, concepts], may be produced by action research. Theory may be generated and refined, and its general application explored through the cycles of the action research process.

- to develop a plan of action to improve what is already happening
- to act to implement the plan
- to observe the effects of action in the context in which it occurs
- to reflect on these effects as a basis for further planning and subsequent action, through a succession of cycles

The CRASP model

More recently a critical action research model, CRASP (box 2.2), has been developed and used by Zuber-Skerritt (1996, 85) for professional, educational, management and organisational development.

Box 2.2: The CRASP model of action research for professional development.

Action research is:

Critical (and self-critical) collaborative enquiry by
Reflective practitioners being
Accountable and making the results of their enquiry public.
Self-evaluating their practice and engaged in
Participatory problem-solving and continuing professional development

---

Conclusion

For the action researcher only the approach can be planned in advance; methods and strategies have to be developed in the field of practice. This could be one reason why Webb (1989) suggests that only one change should be introduced at any time and evaluated and modified as necessary. Only when this is established practice should another change be tried.

Academic rigour

Academic rigour in action research design has been discussed at length in the literature. The main issues focus around questions of reliability, validity and generalisability and are due, in part, to the few academics who share the same underlying philosophies and appreciate the value of collaborative research (Meyer 1993a). The debate centres around whether action research is scientific. Action research can be legitimised as science by locating its foundation in a philosophical stance which differs from that used to legitimate positivist science. In positivist science the researcher is the sole possessor of knowledge from which actions will be drawn and the sole originator of actions to be taken on an essentially passive world. Susman and Evred (1978) assert that extraordinary precautions are undertaken in many controlled experiments; such procedures are at variance with taking action within a social system where human beings react to the researcher as another human being rather than as a researcher per se.

The perceived lack of scientific rigour in action research (Sheehan 1986), owing to its apparent antithesis to truly experimental research (Cohen and Manion 1984), is challenged by Winter (1989), who believes that the researcher needs to adopt a different conception of rigour from that which characterises positivist research. There is increasing recognition of the inappropriateness of (just using) the term 'validity' within a critical action research context, as it simply reflects a concern for acceptance within a positivist framework for research (Kincheloe and McLaren 1994). More appropriate is the term 'catalytic validity', as described by Lather (1991), which points to the degree to which research moves those it studies to understand the world and the way it is shaped in order for them to transform it. Webb (1991) believes that the use of triangulation will enhance validity of the data. Waterman (1998) advocates an active search for opposing perspectives and the movements between theory, research and practice, multiple researchers and methods.

A lack of a general application is not perceived as a problem because a unique, individual situation is being studied, but some findings may be generalisable to other similar settings (Webb 1993). Guiding principles from one study can inform the next action research project. A most significant method to judge the quality of the research approach is thought to be the reflexive accounts by the researcher (Winter 1989, Webb 1991, Waterman 1998):

> It follows that action researchers should also be reflexive about how they create and construct their reports. They should consider how they have framed their work and what led them to their interpretations. (Waterman 1998, 104)

Action research approaches for nurse-led change and development

The definition of action research above (box 2.1) encompasses the seven criteria that Hart and Bond (1995) identify as distinguishing action research from other methodologies (see table 2.4). The authors explicate the seven characteristics from the literature and from an analysis of their personal research. Five studies are provided that demonstrate these criteria:

- micro-politics of action research at a district general hospital
- from sister/charge nurse to manager - empowerment through a staff development programme
- working across professional boundaries and with older people in the community
- progress and procrastination - using a project group to implement changes in service provision for people with disabilities
- changing medication practices in a home for older people

These studies capture the essence, uniqueness and diversity of action research, but they also demonstrate issues of personal and stakeholder power and control within empowering and disempowering organisational cultures. The criterion 'exploring and exposing political dimensions of organisational culture, power and control' has therefore also been included in table 2.4.

Different approaches to action research are found in the literature and can cause confusion. Holter and Schwartz-Barcott (1993, table 2.5) provide a useful overview. Note the similarity with table 2.3 (page 24): classification and characteristics of human interests.

The focus of this book is the use of the critical action research approach, which Holter and Schwartz-Barcott (1993) choose to call the enhancement approach. The focus of their enhancement approach is mutual emancipation (table 2.5) which is reflected in table 2.3 as an emancipatory form of human interest. Both are underpinned by critical social science. It appears therefore that the enhancement action research approach may also be termed 'emancipatory' or 'critical action research' (a more detailed discussion can be found in the following section, 'A useful approach?').

Table 2.4: The criteria that distinguish action research from other methodologies.

ACTION RESEARCH

1. is educative
2. deals with individuals as members of social groups
3. is problem-focused, context-specific and future-orientated
4. involves a change intervention
5. aims at improvement and involvement
6. involves a cyclic process in which research, action and evaluation are interlinked
7. is founded on a research relationship in which those involved are participants in the change process (Hart and Bond 1995, pp 37–38)

In addition:
8. explores and exposes political dimensions of organisational culture, power and control

According to Holter and Schwartz-Barcott (1993) the researcher facilitates the practitioner's discussion of underlying problems and assumptions on a personal level as well as the level of the organisation's culture and the possible conflicts they can generate. The emphasis is on elucidating the underlying value system, including norms and conflicts, which may be at the core of the problems identified. This approach would appear to address the values that underpin nursing and multi-professional practice, the extent to which practitioners identify issues/problems in clinical practice, and the ways in which they may be empowered to effect change in nursing practice.

A useful approach?

Hart and Bond (1995) developed their typology of action research approaches as they believe that the need for a typology arises from the lack of precision in the use of terms, which they state is also an enduring feature of social research and is not a problem exclusive to action research. However, this search for precision could impose constraints on what is essentially a dynamic process within a unique social setting. Rolfe (1998, 195) is critical of typologies that confuse rather than clarify, but Hart and Bond (1995) justify the creation of their typology to 'make sense of what is going on'. Their approaches are labelled 'experimental', 'organisational', 'professionalising' and 'empowering'. They suggest that the experimental and organisational types will be more strongly research-focused, whereas the professional-ising and empowering approaches will be more strongly action-focused. This assertion can be both difficult to comprehend and problematic to

Table 2.5: Characteristics of action research (adapted from Holter and Schwartz-Barcott 1993).

Approaches to action research	Philosophy base	Problem	Focus of collaboration	Theory	Type of knowledge produced
Technical approach	Natural sciences	Defined in advance	Technical	Validation Refinement Deductive	Predictive
Mutual approach	Historical-hermeneutic	Defined in the situation	Mutual understanding	New theory Inductive	Descriptive
Enhancement approach	Critical sciences	Defined in the situation based on values clarification	Mutual emancipation	Validation Refinement New theory Inductive Deductive	Descriptive

put into practice as action and research in this methodology are both interdependent, indistinguishable and inseparable. It is difficult to follow the authors' reasoning as, paradoxically, a symbiotic relationship is clearly evident within their seven criteria (table 2.4).

Critical action research: weak or strong?

A more fundamental approach, previously elicited by Peters and Robinson (1984), would be to describe action research as essentially either weak or strong. Both versions share the following three minimal requirements:

- Involvement-in-change characteristics, i.e. they are problem-focused and directed toward the improvement of some existing social practice.
- Organic process characteristics, i.e. research consists of a series of cyclical or iterative stages of fact finding, reflection and planning, strategic action and evaluation.
- Collaborative characteristic, i.e. research is carried on as a joint, co-operative endeavour among the participants.

The weak version satisfies these three conditions and is not incompatible with other forms of social research. It provides a problem-solving methodology that may be used within a variety of social science perspectives. It does not necessarily entail a commitment to a particular form of explanation of human action or to a particular philosophy of social science. Collaboration will typically take place between an 'expert' and a client group, and the degree of collaboration will be less than total.

A stronger version of action research is described by Peters and Robinson (1984) as a commitment to an underlying philosophy of social science, one with a particular interpretation of the three minimal conditions. The authors' explication of this approach is based on the work of Lewin (1947, 1952) and also of three contemporary action researchers, Elliott (1978), Argyris (1980) and Kemmis (1981). These researchers share Lewin's perspectives but have addressed themselves to questions that go beyond considerations of methodology. They each reject positivist approaches to social reality and embrace instead a belief in the importance of participants' values, beliefs and intentions. They emphasise a self-critical approach to social problems and practices that they feel arise from and are embedded in a social context. They share a concern for marking out action research as an emancipatory form of social research; this implies that, as human beings become active in constructing social reality, they can also act to change it for the better.

Hart and Bond (1995) believe that their typology helps to clarify the complex processes of action research by simplifying them. Yet this could be viewed as a reductionist approach that may have limited value. When initially considering differing (yet often overlapping) action research approaches, the one proposed by Peters and Robinson (1984) offers a more pragmatic and simplified solution to differentiation. The identification of weak and strong versions also provides an awareness of the absence or inclusion of an underlying philosophy of social science. Differentiating between weak and strong versions should enable a more effective analysis of action research studies. The critical action research approach is a strong version as it is underpinned by critical social theory. Before exploring critical social theory, it is necessary to review the somewhat confusing terminology that surrounds critical action research.

Critical action research terminology

Currently three action research approaches are described in nursing literature that share similar characteristics; these are the:

- enhancement approach (Holter and Schwartz-Barcott 1993)
- empowering approach (Hart and Bond 1995)
- emancipatory approach (Grundy 1982; Carr and Kemmis 1986)

According to Lucock (1997), the enhancement approach appears to be a somewhat 'watered-down' version of emancipatory action research, but the difference could lie in the choice of language. For example, she suggests:

> Although Bellman (1996) refers to her project as involving the enhancement approach, it may be regarded as emancipatory in that organisational habits had to be overcome in order to implement patient self-medication and patient-controlled analgesia. It was also emancipatory in that it allowed patients to take charge of their own medication in hospital - something many of them had been doing at home for years! Furthermore, practitioners were also emancipated in that they were no longer influenced by an underlying value system about which they were only tacitly aware. (Lucock 1997, 91)

She acknowledges the work of Habermas as the philosophical foundation for both the enhancement and emancipatory approach. However, the empowering approach (Hart and Bond 1995) does not appear to have an explicit philosophical foundation. Yet uniting all three approaches is the nature of power within the action research process itself. Stringer (1996) notes that the end result (of an action research study) is not so much a transfer in power as a change in the nature of power relations. A key criterion within the empowering approach is the change in power relationships through 'shifting the balance of power' (Hart and Bond 1995, 40). According to Grundy (1982), power in emancipatory action research resides wholly with the group, not with the facilitator and not with the individuals within the group. It is often this change in power relationships that causes a shift from one mode to another (the modes are referred to as technical, practical and emancipatory and reflect the classification and character-istics of human interests and different action research approaches in tables 2.3 and 2.5).

Praxis

Also fundamental to this approach is the operationalisation of praxis that, according to Carr and Kemmis (1986), is the demonstration of shared, congruent values, which result in informed, committed action. This process reflects the view held by Lucock (1997) that the shared values of all involved in the emancipatory approach enable a solution to a problem that feels right and good for the patients as well as for the particular environment. A similar view could be assumed within the description of the empowering approach, as Hart and Bond (1995, 38) also refer to a 'collective consciousness'.

The need for critical action research

Whether critical action research is termed the emancipatory, empow-ering or enhancement approach, it needs to be recognised, understood and enacted in practice settings. It can enhance understanding and start to address 'the frustration, panic and sense of helplessness that drains the profession of motivation, talent, vision and the power to change' (Watson-Druee 1994). However, Meyer and Bateup (1997) cite five action research studies that encountered problems in changing practice owing to issues of power. They suggest that nursing may not be ready for this kind of approach, and that it will be difficult to initiate until there are better working democratic practices in healthcare. Yet issues of power and control are the reality of nurses' professional working lives. Power conflicts exist within almost every healthcare setting, 'where there is an almost constant state of change involving controversy even on a good day' (Nicholson 1992 in White 1998). Nurses need to recognise and understand power issues within their local field of practice, the healthcare organisation in which they work and the political influences that impinge on the organisation and on their day-to-day practice. Where there are problems and evidence for change, nurses need to engage in co-operative and collaborative working strategies, to resolve the issues and effect changes in practice.

The relative powerlessness of nurses was a contributory factor in the action research study undertaken by Waterman et al. (1995). The participants were reluctant to alter the status quo and change practice. They state that the doctors' power was revealed by their needs being given priority over those of the nurses, even when this led to unsatisfactory nursing practice. Street (1995) asserts that it is not very useful to say that doctors have the power and nurses are oppressed by it in the healthcare system, even though all nurses have felt powerless in the face of medical power. Warelow (1996) is critical of nurse-authors who tend to merely describe the dichotomy between medicine and nursing rather than offer any solution.

Senior management power was evident within Hart and Bond's (1995) 'empowering' case study of a staff-development management programme for ward sisters. The management agenda was the creation of an education programme to enable ward sisters to adopt a 'business' ward management role. The sisters were perceived by executive and middle management as traditionalist and culture bound. The authors were faced with what they believed to be a crucial issue for any change agent - 'it may be counterproductive to embark on such collective projects, to establish arenas of empowerment among groups lower down the hierarchy, when these may come into conflict with an individualistic and autocratic organisational culture' (Hart and Bond 1995, 104). Yet, over a two-month period, the authors noted that empowerment emerged through collective work, the creation of trust and openness and through the sharing and exploration of roles as well as actual and potential conflicts.

The value of critical action research appears controversial. It appears that very few studies have currently been undertaken using this approach, and, indeed, there is a dearth of new paradigm research in nursing. Although Meyer and Bateup (1997, 177) have their reservations, they state that, while little of it has been done in nursing, it could be argued that new paradigm research is the most appropriate way forward in developing a body of knowledge relevant to practice. Reed (1995) calls for a framework for nursing knowledge development that is derived from an 'open philosophy' of science, which links science, philosophy and practice. Within critical action research, it is critical social theory which links science, philosophy and practice.

Critical social theory to link science, philosophy and practice

The contemporary philosopher Habermas studied at the Frankfurt School, Germany, where some seventy years ago critical theory is believed to have developed. The theory can be interpreted in many ways. Hammersley (1992) identifies three broadly defined versions of critical theory: the orthodox Marxist position, the Frankfurt School and the feminist position. In spite of differing interpretations, critical theory retains its ability to disrupt and challenge the status quo. Kincheloe and McLaren (1994) believe that it elicits highly charged emotions of all types - fierce loyalty from its proponents, vehement hostility from its detractors. Such extreme reactions indicate that critical theory still matters and cannot be ignored.

Critical theory operates by freeing people from the coercion of ideology through enabling them to recognise the reality of their situation and thereby giving them more control over their own lives. Hammersley (1992) believes that the success or otherwise of a critical theory in bringing about enlightenment and emancipation is a crucial, perhaps the crucial, aspect of any assessment of its validity. His account of the orthodox Marxist's position is that critical theory is the product of intellectuals committed to a revolutionary socialist party. By imparting to the working class an understanding of the nature of capitalist society, and its role in the transformation of that society, a revolution will occur to emancipate all humanity. However, the Frankfurt School did not regard the working class only as an emancipatory force, nor did they see the Communist party as playing a positive role in emancipation. For feminism the abolition of patriarchy is the central concern. These three perspectives reflect, for Hammersley, a diverse audience: for Marx, it was the working class, and for feminists, women. For the Frankfurt School, and particularly for Habermas, the focus appears to be all humanity, although, the overriding concern, according to Carr and Kemmis (1986), is to emancipate people from the positivist 'domination of thought' through their own understandings and actions.

In an interview the philosopher Foucault (Rabinow 1991 in Alvesson and Willmott 1996, 169) reveals his admiration for the Frankfurt School:

> I realised how the Frankfurt School people had tried
> ahead of time to assert things that I too had been

working for years to sustain ... When I recognise all
these merits of the Frankfurt School, I do so with the
bad conscience of one who should have known and
studied them much earlier ... if I had read those works
earlier on, I would have saved useful time, surely: I
wouldn't have needed to write some things and I would
have avoided certain errors.

The central aims of critical theory have been to reassess the
relationship between theory and practice in the light of the criticisms
of the positivist and interpretive approaches to social science, which
have emerged over the last century, and to transform consciousness
(Carr and Kemmis 1986). Habermas (1972, 1974) explores this
process, which resulted in the development of his critical social theory
for changing practice in the world, to enable the self-emancipation of
people from domination.

According to Habermas (1974), the goal of the critical social theory is
an active reflective stand that includes changes that are emancipatory. The
fundamental aim is to expose the contradictions, oppressions and power
imbalances that inhibit individual freedom and autonomy. It entails
analysing power relationships and addressing the dialectical relationship
between theory and practice. A critique of the context of practice, and its
status quo, is undertaken and possible alternative actions considered.

It is interesting to note that in the USA in 1989 Stevens had
proposed that nurses adopt critical social theory (table 2.6) to enable a
critical social reconceptualisation of their environment. She believed
this theoretical approach could enable nursing to increase the potential
for emancipatory change for oppressed communities. More recently
Kim and Holter (1995) also direct the American nurse towards a model
of emancipatory nursing actions with patients, which incorporates the
theoretical framework of Habermas. However, none of these authors
identifies how the use of Habermas's approach could be equally worthwhile for nurses themselves.

Habermas's theory of communicative action

The significance of the work of Habermas is being met with increasing
interest within the nursing literature (see below). Yet, according to Carr
and Kemmis (1986), one of the most persistent general criticisms of
Habermas is his failure to offer a detailed clarification of the epistemolog-
ical basis of his critical social theory. In particular, he has not explicated
his criteria of rationality in terms of which emancipatory knowledge
generated by a critical social theory could be validated or rejected.

Table 2.6: The assumptions, concepts and propositions of critical social theory.

CRITICAL SOCIAL THEORY (Stevens 1989)

Assumptions
- All research and theory are political, in that the social, economic, and political processes of a society are reflected in the microcosm of scholarly investigation.
- Oppressive, structural relations pervade modern industrial society; they usually function automatically, are taken for granted and remain unexamined.
- Mythical, religious, scientific, practical and political interpretations of the world are open to systematic questioning and critique.
- Social conditions are not interpreted as natural and constant but are rather viewed as created by specific historical situations.
- Understanding of the changing conditions of human suffering can be gained through a historical study of the development of oppressive arrangements in society.
- Liberation from oppressive structures is an indispensable condition of the quest for human potential, completion and authenticity.

Concepts
- *Oppression* and *domination* are used interchangeably to indicate unequal power relations embedded in basic structures and functions of society: oppression, which inheres in the social structuring of life limitations that are not equally experienced across groups, is the systematic abbreviation of possibility by which dominated persons are consumed in their quest for human potential.
- *Liberation* is freedom from the coercion and constraint of oppressive social structures; the particular freedom of individuals is understood within a social and collective context.
- *Dogma or ideology* is a dominant, authoritative system of ideas whose underlying assumptions and premises have not been sufficiently examined or challenged.
- *Critique* is a process that consists of several components: (a) oppositional thinking that unveils and debunks oppressive ideology by explaining the implicit rules and assumptions of the historical, cultural, and political context, (b) reflection upon the conditions that make uncoerced knowledge and action possible, (c) analysis of the constraints upon communication and human action and (d) dialogue.
- *Dialogue* is a mutual interaction that raises collective consciousness by clarifying, affirming and integrating the historical, social, political, and economic experiences of communities.

- *Conscientisation* is learning to perceive social, political and economic contradictions and conceiving of ways to take action against oppressive contradictions.
- *Action* is informed, deliberate, meaningful behaviour and verbalisation by those experiencing oppression that seeks to bring about social change; it is based on critical insights, reflection and dialogue.

Propositions
- The greater the distortion between dominant ideology and the reality of people's experience, the more vulnerable is the social system to critique.
- Critique of structural domination that illuminates relationships of power and exposes the unnatural and inharmonious character of existing oppressive relationships potentiates the process of liberation.
- Critical social theory serves to enlighten persons and groups regarding the positions they occupy and the prevalent interests that are served. If persons recognise themselves in the critical interpretations offered, they are conscientised.
- Informed by critique, conscientised persons engage in dialogue with one another and reflect critically upon their own situations with respect to oppressive environments. They take context-specific action to bring about social change based on this critical reflection and dialogue. This liberation process can be conceptualised as dialectical, in that action prompts further reflection and dialogue, which in turn generates renewed action.
- Action for change emanates from groups and communities. Their reflection and dialogue consider (a) their common interests, (b) the risks they are willing to undergo, (c) the consequences they can expect and (d) their knowledge of the circumstances of their own lives.
- The ultimate goal of critical social theory is to facilitate change in structural conditions that (a) distort or inhibit communication, (b) limit life options, (c) constrain action, and/or (d) impose unequal economic, gender or racial imperatives. Social change is advocated so that persons might enjoy authentic existence free from these oppressive conditions.
- Critical social theory is concerned with the reasons and circumstances under which members of societies collectively mobilise to transform the conditions that thwart their full realisation of individual and collective possibilities.

Habermas's reponse has been to develop an analysis of language and argue that the normative foundations that justify critical social theory as a viable and rational enterprise can be derived from an analysis of ordinary language (speech and discourse). His theory of communicative action is an ethical theory of self-realisation that transposes the source of human ideals onto language and discourse (Carr and Kemmis 1986). The political theory rests firmly on the idea of rational communication (Habermas 1974) in which decision-making is guided not by considerations of power but by the rationality of arguments for different courses of action. Communicative action is the collaborative dynamic by which participants come to an understanding with one another. Based on mutual understanding, participants are able to co-ordinate their actions to initiate goal setting and goal-directed action (Rasmussen 1997).

The theory is quite complex, but, according to White (1988), Habermas is asking: what precisely is the contribution of ordinary language to the co-ordination of action, which is necessary for the very possibility of social life? Habermas is concerned with 'systematic distortions of communication' (White 1988, 117). He believes that a way to overcome these is for speakers to orientate themselves towards understanding, i.e. engage in communicative action. Their speech acts must raise, and they must be accountable for, four rationality or validity claims: understanding, truth, sincerity and legitimacy of the speaker.

The 'ideal speech act'

> Only if a speaker is able to convince her/his hearers that her/his claims are rational and thus worthy of recognition can there develop a 'rationally motivated agreement' or *consensus* on how to co-ordinate further actions. (White 1988, 28)

This approach, called the 'ideal speech act', should enable democratic discussion in an environment free from the threat of domination, manipulation or control. Indeed, the goal of communicative action is an interaction that terminates in 'the intersubjective mutuality of reciprocal understanding, shared knowledge, mutual trust and accord with one another' (Habermas 1979, 3), the basis of collaborative practice.

Habermas's theory in practice

Although Habermas's philosophy and subsequent theory still require considerable development, Carr and Kemmis (1986) find his linking of truth and social justice compelling and appropriate for the contemporary development of educational theory. The insight of these educationalists is authenticated by Duffy and Scott's (1998) exploration of the theory-practice gap in nurse education. The authors discuss how they explored a nurse education problem through 'a critical lens' using concepts from Habermas's theory: critical reflection, communicative competence and the ideal speech situation. This led them to consider purposeful action - praxis. Using the theory enabled new insights into an 'everyday' issue regarding (in this instance) the assessment of a student nurse in clinical practice. Undertaking an exploration of the balance of power that existed between a clinical link teacher and staff nurses resulted in the identification of a (familiar) way forward:

> This will involve both educators and clinical staff reflecting
> on this issue collaboratively, with a view to agreeing a
> pathway to change. (Duffy and Scott 1998, 189)

Criticisms of Habermas's theory

Habermas's critics include Fay (1987), whose fundamental criterion for a critical social science is that it is simultaneously scientific, critical, practical and non-idealistic. The main criticisms levelled against Habermas's critical social theory are that it has no bearing on actual political life, is academic and utopian, and that Habermas does not discuss how to put his theory into practice. Ray (1992) refers to the need to address cultural diversity and language difficulties regarding the ideal speech situation. Giddens (1985) states that Habermas's theory is a grand theory, whose concepts are abstract and general. However, the concepts that have resulted from his more recent thinking are being 'tested' in practice (for example Duffy and Scott 1998). The critical action research approach would appear to bring about the theory in practice. Yet McKernan (1996) is highly critical of a grand-theory perspective for action research methodology:

> No action research can be liberationist or emancipatory by
> imposing a grand theory from above. (McKernan: 260)

This view could be persuasive; it appears to reflect the use of grand theory in a prescriptive way. Yet, interpreted within a new paradigm approach, grand theories may provide critical insights for under-standing and changing practice. The interpretation of the theory's concepts should be individualised to the unique situation being studied. Increasingly, there are examples within nursing literature of the use of Habermas's theory as a guiding framework for practice. Heslop (1997) refers to Habermas as most prominent and influential in nursing scholarship. Criticism of Habermas has not deterred nurse researchers (Fleming and Moloney 1996), nurse educators (Hendricks-Thomas and Patterson 1995, Owen-Mills 1995, Wilson-Thomas 1995) or nurse academics (Kim and Holter 1995, Meleis 1997) from valuing his work. A Habermasian approach is now advocated to put nursing on the path to becoming more politically active and powerful and to emancipate nurses within the multi-professional team. Manley and McCormack (1997) consider the potential of his work for exploring the role of the expert practitioner. Warelow (1997) supports the need to focus Habermasian critical theory in terms of conceiving nursing as a form of praxis, thereby concentrating on the emancipatory aspect of his theory. Fulton (1997) believes that one way to promote praxis is to use and teach critical social theory. What is also required to put the theory into practice is an understanding of peer and multi-professional collab-oration, and the role of facilitation.

Collaboration

There is an assumption that healthcare professionals collaborate to provide quality healthcare. This may be the exception rather than the rule, although there is a wealth of published literature exploring collab-oration within healthcare settings and between healthcare staff. The need to advance collaborative practice has been clearly delineated by Wilson (1997), see table 2.7.

These social and political determinants (table 2.7) reflect social policy and subsequent strategic planning; yet there is a dearth of infor-mation on the operational processes required. Wandel and Pike (1991, in Coeling and Wilcox 1994) note that collaboration is a much-discussed but difficult concept to realise. Reason (1995, 1) cautions:

> While co-operation, collaboration, participation are all doubtless 'good things', I suspect that many of us are unclear as to what they might *really* mean.

Collaboration is now on the political agenda. The Government has recognised 'the intrinsic strength of decentralising responsibility for operational management' (Department of Health 1997, 12). This

Table 2.7: Social and political determinants for advancing collaborative practice (Wilson 1997).

- Integrated quality care
- Research/evidence-based practice
- Increasing health expectations
- The Patient's Charter
- Demographic changes
- Technological changes
- NHS reforms
- Health of the Nation
- Strategies for healthcare
- Reprofiling of skill mix
- Educational changes
- Patients' increased expectations
- Working in a more litigious environment

would suggest that any guidelines to be developed for the operationalisation of collaboration in healthcare settings must be devolved to local organisations.

Defining collaboration

There are differing views of the concept of collaboration. An elementary definition of collaboration could be 'working together to achieve something which neither agency could achieve alone' (Ovretveit 1997). Yet, as collaboration is a complex phenomenon, a more detailed perspective, from a concept analysis, is provided by Henneman et al. (1995). Nine specific attributes of collaboration were extracted from the literature:

1. joint venture
2. co-operative endeavour
3. willing participation
4. shared planning and decision-making
5. team approach
6. contribution of expertise
7. shared responsibility
8. non-hierarchical relationships
9. power is shared and is based on knowledge and expertise rather than role or title

In political terms collaboration is linked to cost-effectiveness; collaboration is promoted as the strategy of choice for helping communities and workers adjust to doing more with less. Businesses, governments and philanthropic funders are reinforcing this message by increasingly requiring new kinds of 'teamwork' in the workplace and collaboration among service providers. In the United States results include highly complex innovative service changes. Yet few organisations engaging in collaboration seem willing to seriously question the power relations involved. The status quo remains untouched:

> Transforming power relations is viewed by most public and private funders of collaboration as outside the boundaries of depoliticised change; that is, change that does not raise fundamental questions about or take direct action on issues of political inequalities. (Huxham 1996, 25)

This caution is of significance when interpreting contemporary political views of collaboration. Yet reference to collaboration by the Department of Health (1997, 51) does identify a potentially empowering process:

> Involving staff in service developments and planning change, with open communication and collaboration, is the best way for the NHS to improve patient care. In the future, NHS Trusts will be expected to be open with and involve their own staff. Open communication, including early discussion of any changes, is part of good management, and *all staff* should have greater opportunities to contribute their ideas for service improvement.

Results of collaboration

The political agenda identifies improved patient care as an outcome of collaboration. Other positive consequences cited by Henneman et al. (1995) include:

- the development of a supportive and nurturing environment with improved productivity and effective use of personnel
- increased employee satisfaction
- interprofessional cohesiveness

Collaboration in practice is also seen to enhance confidence, self-worth and importance. It promotes a win-win attitude and a sense of success and accomplishment. To enable the achievement of these outcomes, the process of putting the concept into practice needs to be explored, particularly within healthcare settings.

The advice provided by American nurses Coeling and Wilcox (1994) is to recognise that collaboration between all healthcare professionals takes time and that new skills may have to be learned. The authors' description of collaboration as a style of communication seems to closely resemble Habermas's ideal speech act (see page 40):

> A style in which a person presents and defends his or her own position on issues while disagreeing with the positions of others. This style involves repeated back-and-forth exchanges of ideas ... the verbal give and take that occurs as two or more individuals talk together in an attempt to reach agreement. (Coeling and Wilcox 1994, 46)

The authors undertook a survey of nurse-physician communication concerns to which 180 nurses and 90 physicians responded. The outcome of the survey revealed communication styles linked to gender rather than differences in role and professional status (most of the nurse respondents were female and the physicians, male). For example, physicians tended to focus more on content/tasks, while nurses focus more on relationships. Physicians wanted others to be friendly towards them and yet wanted to maintain some distance between themselves and others. The survey also reinforced previous research findings that, in general, reflected women's need for involvement, intimacy and connection (rapport-talk), and men's independence, status and hierarchy (report-talk).

Requirements for collaboration

In order to initiate collaboration the following antecedents identified by Henneman et al. (1995) should also be considered: identifying an individual's readiness to collaborate, an understanding of one's own role and expertise, confidence in one's ability, excellent communication skills and respect and trust for collaborative partners. An exploration of the contextual factors is also required (table 2.8). The ideal may be far removed from the reality. Nevertheless, the need to develop and promote a positive working context should become clearly evident through participation in a critical action research study.

Table 2.8: Contextual requirements for collaboration (Henneman et al. 1995).

Visionary leaders supportive of autonomy
Recognition of the boundaries of one's discipline
A team orientation with effective group dynamics
Organisational values which include participation and interdependence

As the study of collaboration is in its infancy (Henneman et al. 1995), new patterns of behaviour and team interaction have to be learned. Shared power through collaboration should be possible for nursing despite hierarchies that might reinforce traditional power relations. However, shared power did not appear to be significant within Gueldner and Stroud's (1996) exploration of nursing's twenty-year struggle in the United States to become a credible partner in collaborative research. The authors did not clearly define the concept of collaborative research. There is no mention of action research approaches. Indeed, one of their cited 'successful' examples demonstrated the disempowering process of nurses as task-orientated data collectors undertaking positivist research:

> Nursing's primary contribution to the study is the clinical
> focus and the expertise in collection and management
> of blood samples. (Gueldner and Stroud 1996, 61)

Repetitive themes can be identified in the literature but with a more positive emphasis. For example, Fitzpatrick (1997), reflecting on the power of politics and partnerships in nursing, asserts that collaboration in practice will require the utmost confidence and belief in our own professional identity. Robinson (1997) believes that *understanding* this oppressive state of affairs could nevertheless be a *liberating experience* for nurses. From a traditional position of subservience, nurses can turn the tide and through collaborative partnerships realise their own potential and power. Yuen and Owens (1996) believe that this can be achieved through participatory and collaborative processes such as action research. However, collaborative practice, according to Hickey et al. (1996), is largely misunderstood and rarely valued by academic institutions.

The need for collaboration

The extent to which collaboration is valued within healthcare settings is still to be seen. However, experienced, knowledgeable and confident nurse leaders are required to initiate and sustain collaborative practice. All nurses should recognise their ability to be leaders, particularly in practice settings. Klakovich (1994) discusses connective leadership, which she believes will effectively address healthcare reform while preserving caring practice. The outcomes of connective leadership are identified as: a caring, professional practice environment with empowered nursing staff, collaboration among healthcare disciplines and an increase in the contributions that nursing makes to healthcare policy and delivery system changes. Klakovich (1994) equates the qualities of connective clinical nursing leaders with those of effective change agents. These leaders have mastered interdependence by creating strategic alliances, discouraging competition and encouraging co-operation among all stakeholders in the change process. This approach to leadership complements the thirteen attributes that demonstrate effective and empowering leadership (Wheatley and Smith 1995):

1. an attitude of constant learning rather than assumed mastery
2. the development of high self-esteem
3. willingness to ask questions and listen to answers
4. a capacity for building relationships
5. appreciation of other people
6. ability to develop leadership in others
7. capacity to handle criticism by listening and drawing out concerns
8. innovation and initiative
9. capacity to develop a vision of the future
10. ability to communicate well at every level
11. integrity and trustworthiness
12. capacity to trust others
13. coaching and counselling skills

Leadership potential is within all of us. It will increasingly hinge on relationship-building, being willing to create dialogue and recognising that values will describe the parameters for initiatives and strategy (Malby 1997). A key process to enable intraprofessional and multiprofessional collaboration is that of facilitation.

Facilitation

There is now a greater focus in the nursing literature on collaborative change and facilitation, with educators, managers and practice developers identified as potential facilitators. Burrows (1997) analyses the concept of facilitation for nurse educators. Her study is supported by literature from physiology, psychology, sociology and colleagues' personal perspectives. The attributes that emerge from the literature are:

- genuine mutual respect
- the development of a partnership in learning
- a dynamic goal-orientated process
- the practice of critical reflection

Consequently, nurse educators who facilitate partnerships in learning should also recognise that they have the ability to facilitate partnerships in research. The recognition of transferable knowledge should enable the facilitation of innovative research and development within clinical practice by nurse educators. Indeed, a study by Acharya (1994) identifies this need for nurse educators in practice.

The need for facilitation

Acharya undertook a descriptive, exploratory study of 63 (from a sample of 100) nurses' perceptions of continuing professional education and the need for a facilitator in the clinical area. She found that 52 nurses indicated the need for a facilitator, with nurse educators as the first choice, followed by ward managers. The nurses identified the need for a facilitator to be available during the day and at night, to attend staff meetings, be in possession of a specialist post-registration qualification and be allocated time for discussion on the wards. Burrows (1997) identifies four antecedents for nurse-educator facilitation to become a reality. Unfortunately, they are only narrowly defined. The four antecedents encompass two people or more voluntarily participating, an acknowledgement of learning through facilitation rather than teaching, the facilitator possessing interpersonal skills and being self-aware and that the two people or more understand facilitation. The most significant omission is any reference to a supportive context in which facilitation is to occur and flourish.

Davidhizar (1994) provides guidelines for managers to move away from autocratic techniques and adopt a more participative role for the empowerment of the employee. His advice regarding facilitation encompasses practising active listening, communicating genuine interest and concern, and providing adequate information. Yet neither this advice nor the concept analysis (Burrows 1997) provides any real indication of the extensive developmental process that is required. Torbert (1976 in Reason 1995, 6) believes:

> One must go through an unimaginable scale of self-development before being capable of relationally valid

action. At the same time it is not possible to be perfect, and the facilitator's power is to be essentially vulnerable.

Requirements for facilitation

Reflecting on this advice enabled Reason (1995) to identify the attributes of a critical facilitator:

- they should have the ability to hold and articulate a vision of a future state
- invite others to reach towards it with them
- know that as they do this their actions are in the service of others
- take authority in order to honour and enhance the self-directing capacities of others
- know that as they take authority they will be most severely challenged
- at times be required to let go of their own vision to allow space for the multiple visions that may develop within the community

This advice can certainly assist the critical action researcher to focus on the dimensions of the facilitator role. Yet it is very challenging advice as it possesses intuitive and intangible qualities that are difficult to define.

The process of facilitation in action research is described by Soltis-Jarrett (1997). She identifies four 'philosophically grounded steps' to be considered when facilitating action research:

1. creating a transformative milieu in the groups to provide a structure, authority and rigour
2. illuminating reality to uncover the discourses in the group, in nursing and in society
3. promoting resistance and accepting rejection, because all action (behaviour) has meaning
4. reclaiming reality to maximise reciprocity, theory building and validity

These four steps may be considered useful and should enable a wider appreciation of the action research facilitation process. However there are some significant problematic issues.

The creation of a transformative milieu refers to identifying the practical problems highlighted in the group within the action research spiral. Within this 'philosophical step' there are some noteworthy points. It is recommended that meetings should not exceed two hours, as the co-researchers can get tired and anxious. Also, meetings should not be held at fortnightly intervals or more, as the process can get lost or lessened. One cannot always be so prescriptive when undertaking clinical action research. A flexible facilitator is required who acknowledges that patients' needs may take priority over pre-arranged meetings. Soltis-Jarrett (1997) recommends that the facilitator negotiates with the group the length (and occurrence?) of the meeting. Yet, in reality, it is preferable that 'protected time' for staff is negotiated initially with a senior manager.

Soltis-Jarrett (1997) also directs the facilitator to 'initially enlighten the participants (co-researchers) about their unrecognised social constraints so that they can then identify ways in which they can free themselves from their oppression'. This process is certainly fundamental to critical action research. However, there is an assumption that the facilitator is actually aware of the social constraints and that the co-researchers are unaware of their own situation. While both these assertions may prove correct, and indeed have been highlighted in the literature, the reverse may actually be true. Facilitation of a collaborative approach to exploring social constraints is required.

Illuminating reality, the second step, involves the use of questions to explore 'why do we do what we do?' While there is detailed explanation regarding the need to identify social and institutional practices that oppress and confine individuals, no reference is made to the facilitative use of group reflection on practice. The third step that Soltis-Jarrett (1997) proposes is more problematic. The author is called a Clinical Nurse Specialist (Psychiatry) but states that she practises as a psychotherapist. *The examples of facilitation within the third step* reflect the direct transfer of psychotherapy skills to the action research process. The focus is on the individual with, according to the author, a need to promote resistance. Resistance is perceived as a catalyst for action whether it is expressed as an emotional response (anger, hurt, disappointment) or as an intellectual response. While these responses may emerge within the action research process, a more worthwhile facilitative strategy would be to put into action the concept of praxis (see page 34). This process provides the opportunity for enlightenment and empowerment of both individuals and groups. *The fourth step* also presents some difficulty. The critical action researcher should preferably be facilitating the process of changing reality, rather than, as proposed by the author, reclaiming reality. Finally, but of prime importance, there is no reference throughout the entire article to the use of the change and facilitation process to enhance patient care.

Moving forward - overall objectives of the research

The first two chapters of this book provide critical insights into the knowledge required to undertake nurse-led change and development in clinical practice and a justification for the critical action research approach. The research study enabled an exploration of the process and outcomes of nurse-led change and development undertaken within two hospitals in different NHS Trusts. The research had five primary objectives:

1. To systematically explore with surgical nurses the process of change within the clinical setting.
2. To identify problems within the change process.
3. To determine how innovation and the change process is perceived by surgical nurses, patients/users, managers and the multi-professional team.
4. To explore the role of the 'insider' and 'outsider' action researcher.
5. To identify the outcomes of the change process for patients/users, surgical nurses, managers, the multi-professional team and NHS Trusts.

Critical action research is the appropriate methodology for the study. From a personal perspective, and from a growing literature which increasingly endorses the new research paradigm, the need to undertake collaborative research with healthcare colleagues and patients remains fundamental to my values and beliefs as a nurse, researcher and educator. Adopting a critical action research approach was part of a developmental process for my colleagues and me. I anticipated that it would help nurses to appreciate their own self-worth, understand the forces that impinge on their expertise, professional judgement and development and acquire the appropriate knowledge and skills to effect change in their clinical setting.

Chapter 3
Integrating theory and practice

'Theory offers what can be made explicit and formalised, but clinical practice is always more complex and presents many more realities than can be captured by theory alone.' (Benner 1984)

Development of the first study

The focus for the first study was provided by a group of patients who were reading and discussing the ward philosophy document that was hanging in the corridor of the ward. I was talking to a staff nurse (in my role as clinical link lecturer), and as we walked past the patients they asked us to explain how the Roper, Logan and Tierney (1990) model of nursing helped surgical patients. We talked about focusing on each person with their individual needs and promoting their level of independence both before surgery and following their operation to enable optimum recovery. The patients seemed satisfied with our explanation, but as we walked away we started to reflect on the nature of nursing. How similar was our practice and to what extent did we or any of our peers really apply the theoretical basis of our proposed nursing model (as stated in the ward philosophy) to our everyday practice? To what extent did we believe that the model reflected our practice and how were we putting the concepts into practice? Where was the time to think, reflect and talk about nursing?

Moore (1990) reports on international nursing perspectives for the twenty-first century. She highlights a proactive approach, collaborative initiatives and the need for all nurses to utilise nursing theoretical frameworks for direction in their respective areas of practice. Aggleton and Chalmers (2000, 60) propose that nurses working together should try to assess the contribution that the model makes to their practice. However, no advice is provided on how to accomplish these dynamic proposals. A new model for nursing research, that of action research, has been suggested by Rolfe (1994) with the view to translating nursing theories and models into practice. Chin and Benne (1976 in Girot 1990) had previously suggested that action research could be used not only as a vehicle for change but also to promote the growth and development of nursing knowledge. Informal discussions with clinical nursing colleagues included consideration of how appropriate the RLT model really was for understanding and influencing our clinical practice. The outcome of these discussions was the identification of five objectives to be explored in a critical action research study:

1. To determine how nurses believe they apply the concepts of the model in practice.
2. To identify problems associated with the clinical application of the model's concepts.
3. To investigate the process and outcomes from reflection on practice.
4. To identify patients' perceptions of their care.
5. To assess how innovation based on the model of care is perceived by surgical nurses and patients.

Issues in theory-practice integration

Theory and practice operate in both directions. The relevance of theory to practice is often overemphasised; the usefulness of practice to develop theory is underestimated. Theory helps determine practice, but practice is in itself essential in developing theoretical concepts in nursing. There is a wealth of literature exploring the theory-practice gap. However, Jones (1997) calls for the word 'gap' to be deleted from the nursing language; theory-practice becomes theory practice, or praxis (see page 34), demonstrating that theory and practice share a co-determining interaction that promotes professional growth, development and change through dialogue.

A current educational strategy, which has been adopted for both students and practitioners to facilitate the identification and possible transference of theory-based practice, is that of reflective practice (see chapter 2). Facilitating the use of reflective practice as a means of integrating theory with practice, whether it is in the classroom or a practice area, should be considered part of the lecturer in nursing and practice developer's role (preferably a combined role). There is value in structured reflection (Johns 1993); yet reflection without action may be sterile. Kemmis (1985) argues that reflection is not a purely internal psychological process; it is action-orientated.

Reflective practice within critical action research is an example of how nurses may utilise the critical paradigm (see chapter 2) to promote the integration and development of theory and practice, but they may not recognise the significance of this approach. Keyzer (1985), a nurse tutor, also suggests that without a redistribution of power and control from managers, educators and doctors to practitioners and patients, the implementation of a nursing model would be difficult.

Allen (1985) points out the fundamental aim of critical social theory (which underpins critical action research, chapter 2) is to expose the contradictions, oppressions and power imbalances that inhibit freedom and autonomy. This requires open, unconstrained communication. Speedy (1989) suggests that this approach will not only empower nurses but will enable them to assist patients in making informed choices about their healthcare. Yet there are widely debated views regarding the complex concept of power. Hawks's (1991) definition maintains that power has two main meanings, 'power to' and 'power over'. 'Power over' is a struggle for dominance or to rise from an inferior to a superior position and has a directive force or impact. It encompasses control, competitiveness, authority and (transactional) leadership. 'Power to' relates to effectiveness and includes the ability to achieve objectives, the means of attaining them and the capacity to do so. Power as an interpersonal process involves participation. Within the Roper, Logan and Tierney model (1990, 1996) patient participation is advocated. This can be seen as a collaborative process that involves the 'power to' or potential empowerment of patients by active involvement rather than as passive receivers of care.

Crane (1991) would support the redistribution of power sharing, and she believes that it is educators who provide the climate, the structure and the dialogue to promote praxis (see page 34). She foresees that the purpose of nurse educators, researchers and managers would be to support the nurse clinician so that all are equal nurse practitioners engaged in praxis, and directing the future of nursing.

According to Webster (1990), it is only by involvement in clinical practice that teachers can see whether an innovation or nursing model could actually work. My role in the academic setting enabled me to facilitate learning in the classroom regarding the critical analysis of nursing models and the more theoretically developed nursing theories. Clinical teaching experience enabled me to attempt the deductive process of implementing the concepts of nursing models and theories in practice. At the time no research studies could be found which addressed the extent to which practictioners find the concepts of the Roper, Logan and Tierney (RLT) model of nursing appropriate for patient care. Grossman and Hooton (1993), who acknowledge the need for qualitative methodologies in nursing research, assert that there have been few serious attempts to identify methods of inquiry that could explore unitary concepts at a more informal, clinical level of practice. They advocate the need for a shared conceptual framework, which would transcend university and service structures to shape the model of nursing practice. A significant enabling component would be:

> A college philosophy which considered clinical practice
> to be a worthy part of the nurse teacher's role. (Baillie
> 1994, 155)

Yet the same perspective had previously been addressed by Skidmore (1989), who asserted that education divorces theory from practice by confining it to the classroom - the practical seems less worthy than the theoretical: theory should be experienced in practice, which should also have academic status.

It would appear therefore that to reduce the theory-practice 'gap' and develop nursing knowledge, nurse lecturers need not only to recognise but also to value a collegiate role with practitioners. They need to adopt a collaborative approach to explore the development and use of (for example) nursing models in practice settings. This would entail researching *with* clinical colleagues on a very regular basis, to power share and promote an environment of mutual trust and support. Facilitating reflexive strategies and the implemention and evaluation of the outcomes of individual and group reflection can enable the lecturer in nursing to be instrumental in uniting theory and practice. However Ashcroft and Griffiths (1989) caution that it cannot be assumed that the skills that make effective teachers are sufficient to enable them to facilitate reflective teaching.

Nursing theories and models - controversial and challenging

McKenna defines a nursing model as:

> A mental and/or diagrammatic representation of patient
> care which is systematically constructed and which
> assists nurses in organising their thinking about nursing,
> and in the transfer of their thinking into practice for the
> benefit of the patient and the profession as a whole.
> (McKenna 1989, 762)

The RLT model for nursing was first published in 1980 and has been considered the most popular model in the United Kingdom (UK). Tierney (1998) believes that the RLT model still appears to have relevance even if it is no longer ground-breaking. However, controversy surrounds the nature and application of nursing models and theories (currently there are approximately 40 in total) since their conceptualisation in North America over forty years ago and their subsequent adoption by British nurses in the early 1980s.

The advantages of adopting a nursing model are said to be philosophical, educational, political, professional and managerial. Clark (1982) believes that models assist nurses to organise their thinking about nursing, and contribute to a unique, informed body of knowledge (Ingram 1991). They give direction to practice (Pearson and Vaughan 1986), enhance autonomy and empowerment for nurses (Aggleton and Chalmers 1986, Frissell 1988, M.C. Smith 1990, Chinn and Kramer 1991, Ingram 1991) and enable the evaluation of standards of care and facilitate human resource planning (Kenny 1993). These advantages are presented as conclusions; however, little evidence exists, particularly regarding the RLT model, to support these views.

The implementation of a nursing model in practice challenges traditional ways of working and knowledge development. The philosophical foundation of the RLT model embraces holistic care. Hence the traditional ideology of nursing, assisting the medical role, rooted in the medical pathophysiological model of cure, is challenged. Nurses are encouraged to adopt an individualised approach to care, which focuses on patients' biological, psychological, socio-cultural, spiritual, politico-economic and environmental needs. The changing nature of the nurse-patient relationship to one of partnership is also advocated by the RLT model. A few nurses continue to see medical knowledge and tasks as being in some way superior to nursing (Aggleton and Chalmers 2000). Indeed, the effectiveness of the dominant medical model is still an issue, although Kershaw (1992) acknowledges that medical practice is changing too as doctors are recognising the value of encouraging patient co-operation, independence and self-help. Yet there is continuing reluctance on the part of some nurses to do more than pay lip-service to the value of nursing models to practice (Aggleton and Chalmers 2000).

Tierney (1998) asks whether nursing models are extant or extinct. Problems with implementation in North America are in evidence both from personal observation (study tour) and in the literature. There are areas where their application has been slow or nonexistent (Kershaw

1992), and Huckabay (1991) asserts that American nurses are reassessing the role of models in nursing practice, education, administration and research. This would suggest that the value of these models for practice is still being questioned.

Yet there is a dearth of empirical research both in the US and in the UK relating to nursing models in practice (Silva 1986, Walker and Avant 1988, Fraser 1990). A decade after the RLT model's inception, Fraser asserts:

> It has not been possible to find research which shows
> the validity of the model in practice. (Fraser 1990, 10)

Early researchers who attempted empirical testing of nursing models were, according to Suppe and Jacox (1985), advocates of the 'received view'. Hagell (1989) contends that the logical positivist approach has prevailed despite nursing's contention that it values subjective as well as objective data and is concerned about holistic aspects of care. Yet a lack of any empirical testing of the model would seem justified according to Uys (1987). He argues that models that have their origins in the early 1970s are more philosophical than scientific and that changes identified by different theorists in sequential versions of the models, and based heavily on logical analysis and argumentation, are plausible.

These arguments may be perceived by many practitioners as academic with little relevance for practice. Indeed, according to Tierney (1998), many nurses may have already dismissed nursing models as passé. However, she argues that with increasing scrutiny of nursing's contribution in today's fast-changing world, and the emphasis on multidisciplinary healthcare, the profession is surely as much, if not more, in need of a sense of clarity about what constitutes its own discipline. This perspective may appear alarmist. Yet American nurse theorists (Walker 2001) have published a dire warning to nursing leadership to 'help save the discipline from extinction'. Their ten key unfinished issues, which incorporate Tierney's view, are identified as questions (see table 3.1) and encompass exploring the nature and integration of nursing practice, nursing theory and nursing research. Political considerations are no doubt implicit in these questions. However, integrative questions regarding government healthcare policy and processes and the politics of nursing should be made explicit and cannot be considered in isolation to the future survival of nursing.

Table 3.1: Ten key unfinished issues for nursing (Walker 2001).

- What constitutes the evidence in evidence-based practice?
- What moral, philosophical, ethical, conceptual/theoretical and historical foundations of the discipline are evident in current nursing practices and research?
- Will there be convergence of leadership and scholarship; if so, how?
- What is the interface between discipline and profession and can we put nursing back into clinical practice?
- To what extent are science (theory and research) integrated in nursing; is the integration adequate or is more work needed?
- What is the relationship between scientific and clinical knowledge?
- Is 'theory' part of the other ways of knowing (besides empirics), and what types of theory are important for nursing?
- Who or what constitutes the scientific community in nursing?
- How can we clarify the paradigms of nursing research (types of research)?
- What are the interrelationships and linkages among nursing research, theory and practice, and which comes first?

These issues suggest that nursing has somehow seriously 'lost its way'. Academic and clinical nurse leaders need to recognise, regain and retain the values that underpin caring and compassion for patients and for each other in the political arena of nursing practice, management, education and research. These values should be congruent with the way nursing is managed, led and practised, knowledge is facilitated and advanced in practice and research is undertaken in practice.

Silva and Sorrell (1992) approach the verification of nursing theory through critical reasoning, through description of personal experiences and through application to nursing practice. They suggest that an unsettling dissonance is created between conceptual/research processes and nursing practice and that, in striving for methodological rigour in research in general and theory testing in particular, nurses too often sacrifice their own lived and validated experiences as practitioners of nursing. This approach, and to some extent the key issues (table 3.1), are encompassed within the process, outcomes, practice and theoretical knowledge derived from undertaking the critical action research study.

The Roper, Logan and Tierney model for nursing

The original Roper model was created in 1976. Roper (1976) states that she collated information about 774 patients from 16 general wards, six psychiatric wards and four maternity wards in 12 community districts. The data was collected using a framework based on nursing activities developed by the Nuffield Trust. The study focused on the nature of nursing and where students should practise. Roper identifies nursing requirements common to all patients, whatever their medical diagnosis. However, she does not fully illuminate the process of model development. Nancy Roper teamed up with Winifred Logan and Alison Tierney in 1976, publishing the first edition of the *Elements of Nursing* in 1980. It has been updated four times; the fourth edition was published in 1996. Tierney (1998) maintains that there is nothing in the model which is essentially incompatible with current popular interest in the idea of 'caring' and the ideals of empowerment. The model is grounded in realism and accessibility (Roper 2000). The five key concepts of the model are:

- the dependence-independence continuum
- activities of living (ALs)
- the life span
- the factors influencing the ALs
- individuality in carrying out the ALs

The model for nursing was developed from the premise that, for most people, illness is but an episode in life, and if the same mode of thinking about living and nursing were developed there would be minimal disruption of living while a person required nursing (Roper 2000, Roper and Logan 1985). This statement may be appropriate for many patients with a short episode of acute illness, but how appropriate is it when considering (a) our ageing population and the greater demand for long-term care, (b) the care and support for people with long-term conditions, such as diabetes, eczema, asthma, epilepsy, Parkinson's disease and (c) patients with mental health problems?

Roper et al. (1990, Tierney 1998) acknowledge the influence of the American theorist Virginia Henderson in the development of their model for nursing. According to DeMeester et al. (1989), Henderson (in 1955), through deduction of physical and psychological principles, from the works of Maslow and Thorndike, developed her definition of nursing and 14 basic human needs. Her concept of nursing has indeed acted as a powerful stimulus for many nurses and continues to be cited as a basis for global nursing (Plowes and Fudge 2000).

Borrowed or shared theory that underpins the RLT model includes the concept of human needs within motivational theory, described by Abraham Maslow (1954). An original list of 16 activities of daily living (ADLs) was reduced to 12, in recognition that not every activity was performed daily; dying was added to the original list. To emphasise the active element of their model, all activities are specified as verbs. ADLs are now referred to as activities of living (ALs).

In 1981, Roper et al. published *Learning to Use the Process of Nursing*, which attempted to illustrate how the model could be used as a conceptual framework in the practice of nursing. This in turn led to a project which involved nine practitioners using the model in their practice setting (medical, surgical, psychiatric, elderly care, midwifery, neurosurgery, a diabetic clinic, in district nursing and in health visiting) and writing up their experiences in *Using a Model for Nursing*, (Roper and Logan 1983). The authors state that it was not a systematic evaluation of the model but referred to it as 'a trial of the model in practice'. The outcome revealed that the nurses found the framework both adequate and relevant in the nine settings.

Two significant omissions are identified by Fraser (1990). These are the lack of an identified patient knowledge-base and no critical evaluation of the appropriateness of assessing dependence/independence in the model. There is, however, a dearth of literature on the model's use in practice. Fraser's (1990) literature search found only 17 articles conveying anecdotal evidence (11 on problem identification, two on planning care, four on the implementation of care). Lacking are studies on evaluation of care and nurses' perspectives on the model's usefulness in practice.

The model has been criticised for the use of the ALs as a checklist (Reed and Robbins 1991), the emphasis on the physical aspects of patient care (Cowen 1986, Minshull and Ross 1986, Walsh 1989), and the simplistic nature of the model (Walsh 1991). It is evident that the first two problems indicate an inappropriate adaptation of the model in practice. The model clearly delineates the need to address psychological, socio-cultural, environmental and politico-economic factors which influence the ALs. These factors are cited throughout the Roper et al. (1990) text (Newton 1991). Indeed:

> The addition of politico-economic factors was novel and
> is now indispensable. (Tierney 1998, 81)

Simplicity may be defended as being one requisite of a model capable of being translated into multiple nursing situations (Minshull and Ross 1986). Clarity of language is perceived by Cormack and Reynolds (1992) to represent clarity of thought, and Girot (1990) asserts that the comparatively simplistic nature of the RLT model has developed a common ground for communication between nurse theorists and nurse theorists and practitioners. This would appear to be the case, as Fraser (1990) acknowledges that the model is acceptable to many British nurses and has been widely used in many different practice areas. Parker (1997) acknowledges that the model is easy to comprehend, straightforward and actually works in conjunction with medical practice.

Perceptions within nurse education include the model's continuity for students within diverse clinical experiences (Kilgour and Logan 1985) and the model's flexibility and use in the development of innovative teaching methods (McCaughtery 1992).

Jukes (1988) undertook a survey to identify tools used for the psychological assessment of patients with learning disabilities. He compared use of conventional assessment tools with that of the RLT model. Questionnaires were sent to senior tutors and senior nurses. He concluded that the RLT model was found to be the most popular for a psychologically based skills assessment. The validity of this study is questionable, however, as no details are provided regarding sampling, questionnaire design or analysis of data.

Benner (1984) believes that a model is a tool for use that can guide and clarify practice. Roper, Logan and Tierney view their model as a tool to enhance the analysis of the concepts which contribute to an understanding of the knowledge-base required for nursing practice (Roper et al. 1990). They challenge the academic perspective that criticises the model's theoretical construction:

> We believe that to be useful a model should be readily understood and in the case of nursing, directly relevant and applicable to practice. There is no need for a model to exhaust every aspect of the subject, and, indeed, if its presentation is excessively complicated by detail, its application to practice is unlikely to become readily apparent, however interesting and academically respectable it may be. (Roper et al. 1990, 35-36)

Newton (1991) utilises Fawcett's (1989) framework in her analysis and evaluation of the RLT model and found that the model met many of the identified criteria.

The dependence-independence continuum, a key concept within the RLT model, is central to contemporary perspectives of nursing practice. The focus of independence dominates many aspects of health-care and, according to Masterson (1993), has several dimensions: social independence (which is concerned with having the power to demand rights), economic independence (having the ability to provide oneself with food), physical independence (which involves mobility and being able to take care of one's physical needs) and mental independence (which is about problem-solving, thinking and acting for oneself).

Patient independence is common in many definitions of and descriptions about the nature of nursing. Indeed, Taylor (1993) believes that encouraging patients to find their own level of independence enhances the therapeutic value of nursing. It would also appear to have a social and political significance. As a result of demographic and social factors there is political concern regarding 'the rising burden of dependency' (Allsop 1984). An ageing population places increasing demands on nursing, medical and social services that are already overstretched. Promoting optimal levels of independence could ease this burden, although Watkins (1993) cautions against encouraging independence in older people who are considered mentally and/or physically frail.

Roper et al. (1990) do not provide an operational definition of independence for nursing practice. They believe that the concept is too global to be meaningful. The concepts of independence and dependence are really only meaningful when considered as relative to one another. Indeed, Masterson (1993) concludes that there are both subjective and objective components of the concept. Independence is closely linked to notions of self-worth, self-esteem, dignity and health; a personal sense of control and freedom is intrinsic to independence. However, she also warns nurses against defining the concept too narrowly.

Patton supports these views:

> In programmes that emphasise individualisation of treatment and outcomes, staff may argue, quite justifiably, that independence has a different meaning for different people under different life conditions, it is the unique meaning of the outcomes for each client that should be documented. (Patton 1990, 98)

While Roper et al. (1990, 43) acknowledge, albeit briefly, that there are circumstances where dependence is necessary, they do not appear to acknowledge that some patients seek dependence, especially in hospital where they perceive the caring role of the nurse to be all encompassing. Current Western ideology, however, affirms individual achievement and self-reliance. Nurses could therefore be placed in a somewhat invidious position especially when caring for patients of different cultures who value (inter)dependence and family support. Independence for many Asian women could, for example, result in potential isolation.

The literature pertaining to the RLT model is sparse. Perceptions of the model from nurse educators' and practitioners' accounts have been explored. It would appear that the model has been widely used in the

UK, but the focus on ALs (activities of living) may be to the exclusion of how the other key concepts of the model have been applied in practice. This dearth of information or research regarding the RLT model suggests that there is little value placed on the model or its application to practice. There is potential incongruence between the teaching of the model in an academic setting and its application in practice.

The nursing process

The application of a nursing model in practice is facilitated by the *nursing process*, also an American import. It is a systematic approach to providing individual care. In the US the nursing process continues to be viewed as an appropriate problem-solving process for the twenty-first century (Allen 1997, Alfaro-LeFevre 1998).

Biley (1991) notes that the introduction of the nursing process was perhaps the initial driving force in the rejection of the traditional medical model paradigm. Development of the nursing process was enhanced by the World Health Organisation's (WHO) decision to incorporate it into the programme for nursing/midwifery within the WHO European region in 1983. The widespread adoption of the nursing process in the UK came from the former General Nursing Council in its 1977 revision of the general nursing syllabus. There was significant resistance by British nurses to this initiative, which, in fact, preceded nursing model implementation.

In her literature review Walton (1986) notes that resistance to change is often identified with the implementation of the nursing process. Daws (1988) asserts that its introduction called for a change deeper than a 'simple' change in practice. At that time both the rational-empirical and power-coercive approaches to change (see table 2.2, p. 23) were evident. There was little recognition of the need for nurses to collaboratively explore and 'own' changes in nursing practice.

The Nursing Process Evaluation Working Group (Department of Health 1986) proposed that a study should be undertaken into practitioners' understanding of the relationship between a nursing model and the nursing process; there is no published record of this study taking place. Nurses said that they had always assessed, planned, implemented and evaluated care (the characteristics of the nursing process) and were also suspicious of the new documentation, the nursing care plan, which accompanied the nursing process. This resulted in a spasmodic and haphazard use of the nursing process, nursing care plans and nursing models throughout the UK. Doctors' scepticism was also in evidence. In particular Mitchell (1984) questions the jargon, unnecessary complexity and lack of tested methods of evaluating its use in practice.

Brooking (1988), however, developed a scale to measure the use of the nursing process. 68 nurses were surveyed from eight general wards (four surgical). Face, content and concurrent criterion-related validity were found to be high. The scale was found to have some construct validity. Factor analysis was not undertaken. Test-retest and split-half reliability were found to be high. Brooking asserts that the instrument appears to be reasonably precise, discrete, readily understood, meaningful and comprehensive. Although the scale is not worded as a conventional Likert or Thurstone-type attitude scale, high inter-item correlation coefficients were found. It did not appear that any attempt was made to link the scale with a nursing model to reflect its application in practice, nor is this in evidence in current nursing literature. In fact, Brooking removed three items from the original scale that reflect a holistic approach to care.

Unprepared both professionally and personally for the dramatic changes that challenged their traditional nursing practice, nurse managers, teachers and practitioners were often sceptical of their usefulness. Nurse teachers were instructed to incorporate these approaches into the pre-registration curriculum. Consequently all British nurses who qualified after 1977 supposedly had a theoretical grounding in 'new' nursing practices. The application to practice was, however, limited. Education related to these initiatives for qualified nurses, teachers and managers was virtually nonexistent at that time. The dissonance that I personally experienced, as a then clinical teacher, related to this theory-practice gap. A dichotomy existed between the need to teach the theoretical basis of nursing models, the nursing process and nursing care plan documentation, and any attempt to identify its application and usefulness for patient care in practice.

Nursing care plan

The nursing care plan, the operational tool of the nursing process, is also a controversial issue. Indeed, Walsh (1998) states that some nurses in the USA have now rejected the traditional care plan and moved onto multidisciplinary approaches to care - critical care pathways. Bellman (2000) questions whether multidisciplinary pathways of care when used alone adequately capture the essence of nursing. Alfaro-LeFevre (1998) appears to have combined the use of both in her step-by-step guide.

Nursing care plans are recommended for the benefit of the patient and the nurse. Patients should have access to their care plan to enable understanding and participation in care. For nurses written care plans are tools for providing continuity, communication, co-ordination, individualisation and documentation of professional nursing care

(Bower 1977). They have been used as a teaching tool for students (Daws 1988) and for auditing, peer reviews and staff development (Velianoff 1986). Stevens (1972) earlier noted that any instrument that is supposed to fulfil so many purposes is bound to run into trouble.

Roper et al. (1983) advise nurses to search for simple yet comprehensive documents to reduce 'the complex and time-consuming activity'. However, a study (Reed and Robbins 1991) analysing 52 care plans based on the RLT model in three care-of-the-elderly wards, highlights problems with mobility. The findings reveal inconsistencies in recording problems of mobility, owing to a blurring of the boundaries between the ALs. The problem of within which AL to document a patient problem/need is identified by Walsh (1991). A prescriptive approach appears to negate the creative, innovative, autonomous thinking to which nursing aspires. Yet it should be considered a developmental stage in the evolution of nursing knowledge.

It is difficult to evaluate the Reed and Robbins (1991) study, as there is no clearly stated research question and no cited literature review related to care plan use. Consequently, the authors do not appear to have considered the many variables that Shea (1986) identifies within her conceptual framework to study the use of nursing care plans (table 3.2). The variables encompass:

- nurses' and administrative values
- the environment of care
- structure and function of the care plan
- nurses' education, experience, attitudes and beliefs about nursing
- outcomes of care plan use for the patient, the nurse, the clinical unit, administration and nursing as a whole

The framework is based on value expectancy theory (Lewin et al. 1944) and Becker and Maiman's (1975) model of compliance. Theorists of cognitive motivation often distinguish between two determinants of behaviour: expectancy and value. A positive incentive will motivate more effectively the more it is expected and the higher its value. However, incentives can prove ineffective if they are not valued or are not expected for certain behaviour. Recent researchers have developed this theory which has received extensive empirical support (Roediger et al. 1987). Bellman (1989, 1993) utilises this framework to study surgical nurses' attitudes to care plans and is able to validate the motivating and modifying determinants of care plan behaviour identified by Shea (1986). The framework is also used by Shea et al. (1989) in the implementation of conceptual models of nursing in Canada.

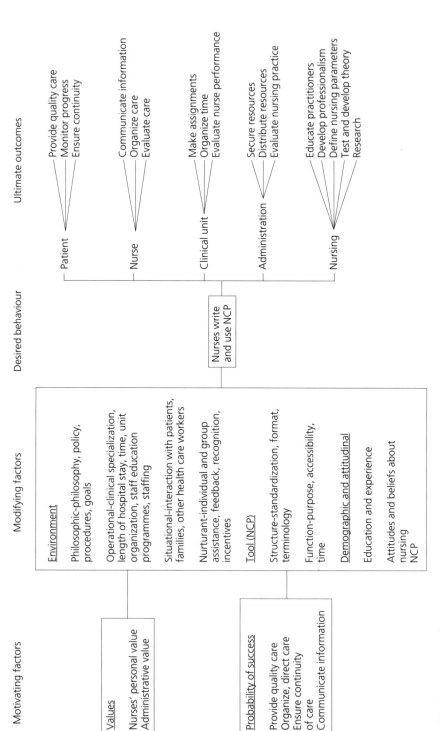

Table 3.2: Framework to study the use of nursing care plans (Shea 1986).

Moving forward

Reed (1995 in Roper et al. 2000) strongly rejects the idea that nursing has matured beyond needing conceptual models for knowledge development and for practice. Aggleton and Chalmers (2000) believe that nurses working with nursing models will be in a stronger position to contribute on an equal footing with other healthcare professionals. What is required, according to Walsh (1998), is a creative, flexible style of working with models, using them as conceptual frameworks and interpreting them as a guide to practice.

In this study, to research the perceived use of a model in practice it was considered necessary to determine nursing process and care plan behaviours and to utilise Shea's (1986) conceptual framework. However, there were other important variables to be considered. These included the extent to which nurses are empowered to implement theoretical initiatives in practice and change strategies to facilitate the implementation and evaluation process.

To initiate the critical action research process a specific problem is identified that is agreed and acknowledged to be valid by all the participants. This enables collaborative strategic action to be planned. Although the key objectives had been identified (page 53), at this early stage I had no idea which problems would become apparent from exploring the use of the RLT model in practice.

Chapter 4
Preparing for the first study

'While doing action research in an organisation is very political, doing research in (and on) your own organisation is particularly so' (Coghlan and Brannick 2001).

The first study was conducted in two phases over a fifteen-month period. Phase one involved selection of the ward in which to undertake the study, feedback of initial findings to the nurse unit manager (NUM) and surgical staff, and collaborative problem identification. Phase two consisted of group reflection and identification of innovations, collaborative planning, implementation and evaluation of these initiatives.

The setting

The objectives for the first study (p. 53) were identified with colleagues within a surgical directorate of a 400-bed hospital, based in an urban location in the southeast of England. The hospital serves a local population of approximately 23,000 people. Patients are admitted to medical, surgical, elderly care, paediatric, acute mental health and intensive care beds. The surgical unit consists of three wards and a day surgery unit; the total number of surgical beds is currently 83. All three wards had a philosophy of care that was underpinned by the RLT model of nursing.

I had worked within surgical settings, in a number of hospitals, for over twenty years. I was known to the nursing staff and the four surgeons of this surgical directorate for approximately six years in my role as lecturer in nursing and clinical link lecturer. I could therefore be considered an 'insider' action researcher. I knew that the RLT nursing model was used throughout the surgical unit; yet, from conversations with colleagues and students, many practitioners and educators (including myself) just paid lip-service to it, used the ALs (activities of living) within the nursing care plans as a checklist and rarely, if ever, took the opportunity to explore the model's conceptual basis in practice, especially from the patients' perspective.

Initial problems of access

As I had worked alongside many of the staff over a number of years I hoped that there was mutual respect, trust and support between us. This was to become evident even before the first phase of the study had commenced as I experienced major problems from both senior management and the ethics committee.

To gain permission to conduct the study I wrote to both the director of nursing (DN) and, at that time, the general manager (GM) of the hospital. The DN appeared enthusiastic but warned me of forthcoming, time-consuming quality initiatives that were due to commence in the surgical unit. The GM was less forthcoming due to concerns regarding increasing nursing workloads and, equally important from his perspective, the study would be of no apparent benefit to the organisation. He therefore refused permission. I felt quite powerless especially as I had not had an opportunity to discuss the study in person. With the support of colleagues in the surgical unit, I contacted the DN again and the quality assurance nursing advisor (who had both apparently been party to the GM's decision) to express my reaction indicating that the King's Fund had provided monies to support the study. Once again, having obtained positive verbal agreement, I went to see the GM to ask him to reconsider. This time he seemed more receptive to the study, possibly by my account of positive outcomes to the organisation resulting from action research that had previously been used in management settings. He asked me to meet with the DN to explore a way forward and subsequently approved of the study, requesting initial feedback in three months' time.

The ethics committee consisted of a senior nurse manager (recently left and position currently vacant), the district pharmacist, a clergyman and five doctors, one of whom was chair of the committee. Although I had prepared a comprehensive research proposal with consent forms for both nurses and patients, I was asked to provide further written information on the RLT model. I was then sent a questionnaire that was difficult to complete, as it was far more appropriate for quantitative medical research. The chair of the committee then met with me to seek clarification and further information. I had originally applied to the ethics committee at the beginning of June. Permission was not forthcoming until the middle of September.

At the time these two ordeals made me angry, upset and frustrated. I tried to rationalise the situation by persuading myself that the delays and queries I was experiencing were valid as they forced me to clarify my thinking. I appreciated that I was asking many people to invest in a high level of risk by agreeing to the study as there was no way of knowing the outcome or even the direction of the action research approach. Nevertheless I felt aggrieved that the nurses who would be directly affected by the study had not been asked (by senior managers) to contribute to the final decision. Meyer (1993a) suggests that it would be difficult for the participants to give informed consent when the nature of the proposed change is unknown and determined by an emerging reality. It would also be difficult for individuals to withdraw, because they are part of a committed group working together for change. In retrospect, I was rather naïve and should have anticipated the problems that I experienced, for I had assumed that the collaborative nature of a nursing research study would have been viewed favourably by non-nurses even if they could not fully comprehend the action research approach or the nature of the RLT model of nursing itself.

All four surgeons were informed of the study. Each was provided with the same written information that had been sent to the ethics committee with the offer to meet personally with them to clarify issues and/or provide further information. Expressions of interest and support were received from three of the surgeons; however, I received an abrupt telephone call from the fourth surgeon. After two attempts at trying to meet with him, I was told that I could not have access to his patients for the study. Once again my nursing colleagues were most supportive. This surgeon's response was perceived as characteristic, and hence we did not use his patients for the first phase of the study. In change-theory terms, this surgeon was a 'late majority adopter' (Rogers 1995). When latterly he heard from his colleagues about the changes and developments taking place, he then requested that his patients should also be included in the study.

Sampling approach

The non-probability sampling approach is adopted within an action research study. Consequently research findings are, in the main, perceived to be non-generalisable. Polit and Hungler (1985) state that, despite this fact, the majority of samples in most disciplines, including nursing research, are non-probability samples. Patton (1990) refers to the logic and power of purposeful sampling, which lies in selecting information-rich cases for study in depth.

> The logic of purposeful sampling is quite different from the logic of probability sampling. The problem is, however, that the utility and credibility of small purposeful samples are often judged on the basis of the logic, purpose and recommended sample sizes of probability sampling. What should happen is that purposeful samples be judged in context - on the basis of the purpose and rationale of each study and the sampling strategy used to achieve the study's purpose. (Patton, 1990, 185)

From the several different strategies described by Patton (1990), the *combination*, or *mixed-purposeful*, sampling approach was felt to be the most appropriate. This strategy permits information-rich cases for in-depth study with the use of triangulation (see page 88) enabling sufficient flexibility to meet multiple interests and needs.

Initial participants

The nurses within the surgical unit bring diverse perspectives to nursing practice, owing to differences in nursing expertise, socio-cultural backgrounds and academic attainment. Their clinical grading at the initiation of the study is depicted in table 4.1.

Most staff worked on day duty, two chose to work on permanent night duty and some staff chose internal rotation. Thirteen staff had undertaken further education in nursing models/nursing process. Seven felt able to apply this knowledge in practice. Table 4.2 demonstrates the system of ward organisation perceived by the staff to be operational in their ward.

Table 4.1: Clinical grading of initial 22 participants (Ward A - includes night sister).

Grade	G	F	E	D
Total	4	3	7	8
Ward A	2	1	2	3
Ward B	1	1	2	3
Ward C	1	1	3	2

Table 4.2: System of organisation adopted in the three wards.

System of ward organisation	*Primary nursing	*Team nursing	*Patient allocation	*Task allocation
Total	–	15	7	–
Ward A	–	8	–	–
Ward B	–	5	2	–
Ward C	–	2	5	–

*The terms were not defined for the respondents. On wards B and C, the nurses were not in agreement about the type of system of organisation used in their ward.

Initial data collection tools

To start to gauge the perceptions of nurses and patients regarding the use of the RLT model of nursing in practice three *data collection tools* were developed concurrently. A nurses' *self-rating scale* on the use of the RLT model in practice (table 4.3) was distributed to participants. The scale was based on an adapted version of the Brooking (1986) scale to measure the use of the nursing process (see page 64), and the additional RLT items (table 4.4) were informed by Shea's (1986) conceptual framework to study the use of nursing care plans (table 3.2). I also interviewed patients regarding their care and perceptions of the concept of patient independence and undertook an analysis of patients' care plans. The patients' *interview proforma* (table 4.5) and the *care plan analysis tool* (table 4.6) were derived from the RLT self-rating scale (see table 4.3).

Table 4.3: Ward nurses' self-rating scale.

	Yes Always Excellent	Yes Usually Good	Yes Often Fair	Some Times Poor	Don't Know	No Never
1. Does the written nursing assessment begin within 24 hours of admission?						
2. Are all the activities of living documented within 24 hours of admission?						
3. Does the assessment tool, based on the nursing model, enable a comprehensive nursing assessment?						

Table 4.3: (contd).

	Yes Always Excellent	Yes Usually Good	Yes Often Fair	Some Times Poor	Don't Know	No Never
4. Are levels of dependence/ independence recorded in the care plan for appropriate activities of living?						
5. Is the developmental stage of each patient considered when planning care?						
6. Are potential problems identified as well as actual problems?						
7. Are problem statements made with the knowledge and agreement of patients and/or relatives?						
8. Are problems numbered and documented according to the appropriate activity of living?						
9. Are care plans produced which incorporate patients' problems?						
10. Are patients encouraged to read their care plans?						
11. Are care plans updated at least once daily?						
12. Are psychological factors addressed within the care plan?						
13. Are socio-cultural factors incorporated into the plan of care?						
14. Are environmental factors identified in the care plan?						
15. Are politico-economic factors highlighted in the care plan?						
16. Are nursing care planning discussions or rounds held in the ward?						
17. Do care plans include discharge planning?						

(contd)

Table 4.3: (contd).

	Yes Always Excellent	Yes Usually Good	Yes Often Fair	Some Times Poor	Don't Know	No Never
18. Are goals (aims of care) incorporated into the care plans?						
19. Do the goals include both long- and short-term goals?						
20. Are goals written in terms of patient outcomes i.e. changes in the patient?						
21. Do goals identify the level of independence to be achieved?						
22 Do goals specify a time for achievement?						
23. Are planned nursing actions included?						
24. Are planned nursing actions agreed upon with patients and/or relatives?						
25. Does the system of ward organisation promote individualised care?						
26. Are nurses allocated to the same patients?						
27. Are care plans used for verbal handover reports?						
28. Does the verbal handover occur at the patient's bedside?						
29. Are nurses responsible for written and verbal reports on their patients?						
30. Do nurses take part in medical rounds for their patients?						
31. Are care plans used at night as a basis for giving care?						
32. Is evaluation recorded on the care plans?						
33. Are dates for the evaluation of patient problems included in the care plans?						

Table 4.3: (contd).

	Yes Always Excellent	Yes Usually Good	Yes Often Fair	Some Times Poor	Don't Know	No Never
34. Is level of independence achieved/degree of dependence (within appropriate activities of living) recorded in the evaluation?						
35. Are patients and/or relatives included in the evaluation?						
36. Are care plans modified according to the results of the evaluation?						
37. Is every entry/deletion on the care plan dated and signed?						
38. Have all ward nurses in the last 3 years updated their knowledge of nursing models?						
39. Is the clinical application of the Roper, Logan and Tierney Model of Nursing taught to students in the School of Nursing?						
40. Do nurse teachers facilitate the clinical application of the Roper, Logan and Tierney model?						

Table 4.4: Derivative of the RLT self-rating scale items and their relationship to Shea's (1986) conceptual framework.

Item	Derivation	Conceptual Framework (Shea 1986)
2. Are all the activities of living documented within 24 hours of admission?	Researcher	Probability of success
3. Does the assessment tool, based on the model of nursing, enable a comprehensive nursing assessment?	Researcher	Tool – function

Table 4.4: (contd).

Item		Derivation	Conceptual Framework (Shea 1986)
4.	Are levels of dependence/ independence recorded in the care plan for appropriate activities of living?	Researcher	Philosophic – policy
5.	Is the developmental stage of each patient considered when planning care?	RLT (1990)	Nurturant
8.	Are problems numbered and documented according to the appropriate activity of living?	Researcher	Tool – structure
10.	Are patients encouraged to read their care plan?	Wright (1986)	Situational
12.	Are psychological factors addressed within the care plan?	Walsh (1991)	Philosophic – policy
13.	Are socio-cultural factors incorporated into the plan of care?	RLT (1990)	Philosophic – policy
14.	Are environmental factors identified in the care plan?	RLT (1990)	Philosophic – policy
15.	Are politico-economic factors highlighted in the care plan?	RLT (1990)	Philosophic – policy
21.	Do goals identify the level of independence to be achieved?	Aggleton and Chalmers (1985)	Philosophic – goals
25.	Does the system of ward organisation promote individualised care?	Schrober (1991)	Probability of success
28.	Does the verbal handover occur at the patients' bedside?	Biley (1989)	Operational

Table 4.4: (contd).

Item	Derivation	Conceptual Framework (Shea 1986)
34. Is level of independence achieved/degree of dependence (within appropriate activities of living) recorded in the evaluation?	Researcher	Nurturant
37. Is every entry/deletion on the care plan dated and signed?	Long (1981)	Accountability
39. Is the clinical application of the Roper, Logan and Tierney model taught to students in the School of Nursing?	Researcher	Education
40. Do nurse teachers facilitate the clinical application of the Roper, Logan and Tierney model?	Researcher	Probability of success

Four 'expert' practitioners, three 'academic' nurses and one clinical nurse specialist, all with a master's degree in nursing, were asked to comment on the tools. A G-grade sister from another unit agreed to trial the self-rating scale. Some rewording of items, and the omission of one item, was suggested. Favourable and enthusiastic comments overall were received. The interview proforma was piloted on two patients. Some minimal adjustments were made following their feedback.

Table 4.5: Interview proforma for patients.

PATIENT INTERVIEW SCHEDULE

1. On admission and over the past 24 hours what did you feel about the information that was written on the assessment part of your nursing care plan?
2. To what extent did the nurse focus on your ability to be independent while in hospital?
3. Do you think that nurses should consider the stage of a person's life (e.g. middle age) when planning care? Why is this important to you?

Table 4.5: (contd).

PATIENT INTERVIEW SCHEDULE

---

4. Have all your problems been recorded in the nursing care plan?
5. Do you read your nursing care plan?
6. How do the nurses help you to cope with anxieties/worries?
7. Have the nurses taken into account your social/cultural needs?
8. Have the nurses taken into account how you will be able to maintain your lifestyle on discharge home?
9. Is a discussion between nurses about your care held at the bedside? How do you feel about this? Are you included in the discussion?
10. Do you know what the nurses are trying to help you to achieve? Do you understand and participate in this?
11. Do you have all the information you need to make decisions regarding your care?
12. Do the same nurses look after you from day to day?
13. Are you or your relatives asked to comment on the nursing care you have received?
14. On a scale of 1–5, with 5 being the most important and 1 being the least important, how would you grade the following:

    Surgical nurses should:

    a) encourage patients to be as independent as possible
    b) consult patients and their relatives, whenever possible, in decisions regarding their care
    c) treat each patient on an individual basis

15. How else can surgical nurses help their patients?
16. What has helped to make you feel more independent while you have been in hospital?
17. Can you suggest how surgical nurses can promote independence in the future?

RLT self-rating scale process

The RLT self-rating scale (table 4.3) was sent to every qualified nurse, day and night duty, in the three wards. An explanatory letter accompanied the self-rating scale with guidance for some of the items and an attached envelope for return. Respondents were assured that there were no right or wrong answers, and a contact number was provided. Also included was a section for any comments participants wished to make. The response rate was 22 (73%). Of these, eight were from A ward, seven from B ward and seven from C ward. Initially 22 staff had agreed

Table 4.6: The Roper, Logan, Tierney Care Plan Analysis Tool.

Ward: ....

	Yes	Insufficient Information	No
1. Does the written nursing assessment begin within 24 hours of admission?			
2. Are all activities of living appropriately documented within 24 hours of admission?			
3. Are levels of dependence/independence recorded in the care plan for appropriate activities for living?			
4. Is the developmental stage of each patient considered when planning care?			
5. Are potential problems identified as well as actual problems?			
6. Are the causes of patients' problems recorded?			
7. Are problems numbered and documented according to the appropriate activity of living?			
8. Does the care plan incorporate patients' problems?			
9. Are care plans updated at least once daily?			
10. Are psychological factors addressed within the care plan?			
11. Are socio-cultural factors incorporated into the plan of care?			
12. Are environmental factors identified in the care plan?			
13. Are politico-economic factors highlighted in the care plan?			
14. Do care plans include discharge planning?			

(contd)

Table 4.6: (contd).

	Yes	Insufficient Information	No
15. Are goals incorporated into the care plans?			
16. Do the goals include both long- and short-term goals?			
17. Are goals written in term of patient outcomes i.e. changes in the patient?			
18. Do goals identify the level of independence to be achieved?			
19. Do goals specify a time for achievement?			
20. Are planned nursing actions included in care plans?			
21. Are care plans used at night as a basis for giving care?			
22. Is evaluation recorded on the care plans?			
23. Are dates for the evaluation of patient problems included in the care plans?			
24. Is level of independence achieved/degree of dependence (within appropriate activities of living) recorded in the evaluation?			
25. Are care plans modified according to the results of the evaluation?			
26. Is every entry/deletion on the care plan dated and signed?			

to participate (table 4.1). More staff had been recruited during development of the tool.

Initially, 16 (53%) questionnaires were returned. Following a reminder letter, the final response rate was 22 (73%). From his review of the literature, Robinson (1989) concludes that a 50%-60% response rate is the best to be expected if no follow-up letter is issued; 65% constitutes a 'fair' return and anything above is very good.

The self-rating scale was analysed using the scoring system developed by Brooking (1986), which revealed that the nurses believed that they applied the concepts of the model well most of the time. Nine nurses believed that they often implemented the model in practice, while the majority (13) indicated that they usually did.

The highest/positive responses were to the following:

- Does the written nursing assessment begin within 24 hours of admission?
- Are problems numbered and documented according to the appropriate activity of living?
- Are nurses responsible for written and verbal reports on their patients?
- Does the system of ward organisation promote individualised care?

The lowest/negative responses were to the following:

- Does the verbal handover occur at the patient's bedside?
- Are politico-economic factors highlighted in the care plan?
- Do goals specify a time for achievement?
- Are environmental factors identified in the care plan?

Patient interview process

Originally, 12 patients were to be interviewed, four from each of the three wards. In practice, however, eight patients were interviewed over a two-month period. This was in part due to pressure of work, which, at that time, only enabled me to visit the clinical areas on one day per week (for clinical teaching/student and ward-staff support). I had no working knowledge of the patients; therefore I identified with the ward staff those patients who were nearing discharge and would be willing to talk to me. Most of the patients had friends and relatives visiting and/or they were too ill to be subjected to an interview of approximately one hour in length. The ages of the patients interviewed ranged from 64 to 82, and they were all between three and five days post-surgery.

I found that I could only interview one patient on each visit to the clinical areas, as although I had devised a semi-structured tool with some open-ended questions (table 4.5) most of the patients wanted to talk further, especially about the whole hospital experience and their plans and concerns about going home. As a researcher I knew that I should encourage the interviewee to focus on my specific questions. However, as a nurse I believed the digressions to be therapeutic and likely to enhance our rapport. On two occasions, at the close of the inter-view, I sought information on the patient's behalf from the ward staff.

In my general introduction to each patient I said that I was a surgical nurse of long-standing and explained how their participation in the study could help the nurses to improve the quality of patient care. I also provided written information and a 'consent to participate' form. Anonymity was assured, and I stressed that any information told to me in confidence would not be divulged. All agreed to participate.

Interviews were taped using a micro-cassette recorder, but a quiet area for the interview could not always be found. Usually, the patient's day room was used, but even with a 'Do not disturb: interview in progress' sign on the door there were interruptions, mainly from inquis-itive nurses. One patient was interviewed sitting in the main corridor. The worst recording was with a patient confined to his bed. However, with the recorder placed as close to the patient as possible, I was able to produce a reasonable recording despite continuous background noise.

At the beginning of the interview I ensured that each patient felt comfortable and offered them a drink. To establish a rapport I spoke with them about how they came to be in hospital, where they lived and how they were feeling. I told them to ask me if they would like a question repeated or clarified. The interview schedule was placed within view of the patients so that, as well as my verbal request, they could also read each question in turn (two of the patients had poor vision). The patient's nursing care plan was accessed and consulted during the interview. The patients said that they did not feel inhibited or intimidated by the presence of the tape recorder, which both surprised and reassured me.

All except one of the patients said they had enjoyed the interview experience and were delighted to have been asked their opinion. One patient, though, recently widowed, on hearing question 8 about returning home became tearful and talked about life without her husband. I had to adopt the role of counsellor and seriously considered abandoning the interview. This also presented me with an ethical dilemma. I had caused the patient pain and distress, yet she did appear to recover after about fifteen minutes; she said that she was glad to have told someone how she was really feeling and then decided to continue with the interview. Holloway (1992) suggests that research interviews can be therapeutic. Reciprocity exists according to Lofland and Lofland (1984). The researcher gains knowledge from the informant who, in turn, finds a patient listener for their thoughts and feelings. This patient was not atypical. Life crises may alter perceptions yet, in context, their perceptions are as valid as patients not experiencing the grieving process.

Transcribing was undertaken as soon as possible following each interview. Each interview was personally transcribed word for word to enable familiarity with the data. The findings were categorised as: patient assessment, patient independence, psychological and socio-cultural needs, patient participation, and patient satisfaction. All but one of the patients had been hospitalised on a previous occasion. The comparisons that they made between past visits and their current stay were most enlightening.

Patient assessment

The findings from the patient interviews would suggest that the benefit of an initial detailed assessment cannot be overestimated, as this incorporates individual needs at a specific stage of life. I had anticipated that the detailed questioning on admission might have been viewed as intrusive by some of the patients. However, all eight of the patients stated that they were asked appropriate information on admission. The initial RLT assessment was viewed positively. It was seen to be reassuring and reduced feelings of insecurity. For example:

> I thought it was very good. They treated you as an individual. Finding out all about me; well, it made me feel more secure really, and I felt I would be well looked after.
>
> I remember the nurse going through all that [activities of living]. I didn't mind a bit being asked all those questions. Anything that I can see that is going to help me is quite all right as far as I am concerned.
>
> I did feel apprehensive. I'm not a brave person. I found it rather comforting that they wanted to know so much about me.

Patients' positive perceptions of assessment were found to be congruent with the findings from the nurse's self-rating scale (page 81).

Promoting independence

The RLT model focuses on the need for nurses to promote an optimum level of independence for each patient within the activities of living. Seven of the patients recognised the nurse's role in promoting independence and believed it to be as important as treating each patient as an individual. One patient remarked:

> *I am independent as much as possible. I would rather get out of bed without any help. Oh, yes, I definitely feel it is important for nurses to encourage patients to be independent. Before when you came into hospital they said to you: 'Into bed', until someone said you could go to the toilet. It's a godsend now. I think you get better quicker. It gives you more confidence. It's certainly better now.*

Ways of promoting independence were described. The psychological benefit of having the right to choose to be independent with the resulting increase in self-confidence was an important issue discussed by three patients.

The need for adequate and continuous pain relief was highlighted. The experience of acute pain was described by half the sample, who stated that pain had reduced their ability to be independent. One patient declared:

> *I am naturally an independent person; so that does not come amiss as far as I am concerned. I appreciate what the nurses are trying to do - to make us do things for ourselves, although, at times, because of the pain, it has been agony.*

There must be appropriate pain relief and a balance between promoting independence to enhance feelings of well-being and reduce the risks of post-operative complications, and ensuring that patients have sufficient rest to enable recovery. Also, four of the patients stated that neither discharge planning nor the ability to be independent and self-caring at home had been discussed with them.

Psychological and socio-cultural needs

Psychological and socio-cultural needs are addressed within the RLT model. Only three of the patients felt that nurses provided appropriate explanation and reassurance. Two patients made explicit that nurses appear to focus on physical needs rather than caring for the whole person. The nurses focused on physical safety, but to the patient psychological safety was perceived as equally important. The physiotherapist was perceived to have more time to spend with each patient and was also seen as knowledgeable and approachable. While the nurses seemed in general to be more concerned with physical needs the physiotherapist appeared to have more time to respond to individual patients' psychological needs. A significant finding was that seven of the sample confided their fears/anxieties to her.

Well, I'll tell you something: there is a very good physio-therapist, and I have a great respect for her. She is a very good psychologist ... Now one thing Mary said to me was, you are going to get better. All right, you do not feel that you are going to get better now, but you will, and I wanted to hear somebody say that to me. She cared about me and the whole treatment, not just the exercises.

I did ask the physiotherapist where it was going to be done. I was just curious how they were going to do it [the operation], and she explained it to me. I suppose I could have asked one of the nurses. Mary is direct, and I suppose positive in what she says.

I told the physio - you know, Mary - at first, but then I was talking to a little nurse the other night; she was telling me things and explaining it all to me, and she put me quite at ease. I felt relaxed.

I felt much more positive once I had spoken to Mary. The nurses seemed to focus on my physical needs.

Seven patients felt that it was very important to discuss their socio-cultural needs. One respondent had a disabled husband whom she cared for:

They put something down [in the care plan] about my husband and social services. That was my main worry - that he was being looked after - and they got the social worker to sort that out.

Two patients specifically referred to feeling positive as an aid to recovery.

The very fact that I could stroll down the ward with all my bottles and pipes ... the first day I got up to walk, that was good; it gave me confidence to know I was doing things for myself - a positive feeling.

Patient participation

Patient participation in planning, undergoing and evaluating care revealed that only half the patients felt they were included in decisions regarding their care. However, not all patients wished to participate.

> *Well, I just thought leave it to them ... they know what*
> *they are doing. I just thought, well, if anything had gone*
> *wrong, then I would have said.*
> *I don't always think we know what is best for the*
> *patients, do we? It is nice to know what is going on, but*
> *I feel that the nurses know best.*

Seeking and clarifying information was undertaken by six of the sample. Of the six patients who complied with the nurses' wishes, only two felt that they had received sufficient information. Three patients and two of their relatives felt inhibited and unable to comment. This did not demonstrate empowerment of patients by providing sufficient information to enable decision-making and informed choices.

Six patients believed that there was continuity of care, and all but one identified a preference for care to be given by the same nurse. Ward A retains each patient's care plan at the bedside, and handovers are conducted at the bedside. Three of the five patients interviewed on this ward had read the care plan; four believed that they needed permission to do so.

> *I have always thought that when those things* [nursing
> care plans] *are there they are for the staff not for us. It*
> *just didn't dawn on me that I could have looked at it.*

> *In the first place I was being nosey. I didn't know if I*
> *should or not. I thought, is anyone looking?* [laughs] *The*
> *nurse said: 'That's all right; you're allowed to read that.'*

> *My goddaughter picked it up, and she read bits of it to*
> *me, but then she read it all the way through because*
> *she is dead nosey. She was really pleased with it; she*
> *said it shows that they are really caring about you. The*
> *nurse did say to me that I could read it. It's much better*
> *nowadays. I would rather know what is going on, and*
> *to be able to read it yourself is very reassuring.*

Four of the five patients liked the bedside handovers and appreciated the involvement in the discussion.

> *What I liked is that, when they change shifts, they*
> *actually come around the bed, and the nurse describes*
> *what has happened, and then they ask you have you*
> *got anything to add. I liked that.*

Most patients indicated that they were becoming increasingly aware of being involved in their care. However, they all said, characteristically, that they would normally not worry the nurses for information, because they appeared to be so busy.

Patient satisfaction

Overall, the patients said that they felt very pleased with the care they had received, and virtually all regarded individual care and patient independence to be the most important aspects of care.

> *I like the freedom to do within reason anything you like. It's a much more relaxed atmosphere now, a lot better.*

> *You know, I am very pleased to have this interview. That's another thing that impresses me - that you have taken the trouble to come and ask me what I think about it all. I have changed my mind completely from when I was in this hospital five years ago.*

Fitzpatrick and Hopkins (1983) caution that many patients are reluctant to express critical comments about their healthcare. However, there is now a focus on and need for greater user involvement. These patient responses were not found to be socially desirable responses but distinct perceptions of personal experience.

The data from the patient interviews was contrasted with the findings from the nurse's self-rating scale and the data from the analysis of the eight patients' nursing care plans described in the following section.

Nursing documentation

Patton (1990) believes that records and documents are a particularly rich source of data, and Schwartz and Jacobs (1979) value secondary data as 'naturally occurring' and subsequently uncontaminated by the researcher. However nursing care plans are not always straightforward reports of activities. Reed (1992) demonstrates the significance of the social context by comparing the care plans on two wards and concluded that it was clearly spurious to assume that a lack of written data indicated a lack of assessment or knowledge, or that what nurses wrote was entirely divorced from their practice. This has implications for my interpretation of the data, hence the decision to employ a multiple-methods approach for phase 1 of the study. This would attempt to address problems of misinterpretation and present a reasonably representative account of the complex world of nursing practice.

The RLT care plan analysis tool was devised in conjunction with the nurse's self-rating scale and the patient interview tool. A care plan analysis was completed immediately following each of the eight interviews. Analysis was undertaken by utilising the simple scoring device adopted by Brooking (1986). Nine of the items scored full marks. These were:

- All the patients receive a written assessment within 24 hours of their admission.
- Potential problems are identified as well as actual problems.
- The causes of patients' problems are recorded.
- Problems are numbered and documented according to the appropriate activity of living.
- Care plans are updated at least once a day.
- Goals are incorporated into the care plan (but see below).
- Planned nursing actions are included in care plans.
- Care plans are used at night as a basis for giving care.
- Evaluation of care is recorded on the care plans.

The items that scored the lowest marks were:

- Psychological factors (addressed in only one of the care plans).
- Both long- and short-term goals (included in only one of the care plans).
- Goals do not identify the level of independence to be achieved (but see above).
- Dates for the evaluation of patient problems (not included in the care plans).

Triangulation of data

There is no clear agreement on the meaning and purposes of triangulation in research. Shipman (1988) states that triangulation is the technical term for two or more methods of collecting data. Denzin (1978) identifies four basic types of triangulation: (1) data triangulation - the use of a variety of data sources in a study, (2) investigator triangulation - the use of several different researchers or evaluators, (3) theory triangulation - the use of multiple perspectives to interpret a single set of data and (4) methodological triangulation - the use of multiple methods to study a single problem or programme. The goal of triangulation in any study, however, is to enhance the validity and credibility of findings because of the weaknesses of any single method. I undertook triangulation of the findings from the self-rating tool, the patient interviews and their nursing care plans.

> Using triangulation is recognition that the researcher needs to be open to more than one way of looking at things. A corollary to this insight is that purity of method is less important than dedication to relevant and useful information. (Patton, 1990, 193)

Triangulation of data is a form of comparative analysis. I attempted to compare the data from the nurses' self-rating scale with the data from the patient interviews and from their nursing care plans. Patton (1990) cautions that the findings generated by different methods do not automatically result in an integrated whole; initially, qualitative and quantitative data often produce conflicting perspectives. Another difficulty is deciding whether the results from multiple methods have converged, which, according to Jick (1983), remains 'a delicate exercise'.

Comparison of the findings from the three instruments revealed the varied dimensions of the perceptions of the application of the RLT model to practice in the surgical unit. Five complementary items were identified (and see table 4.7):

- appropriate written assessment within 24 hours of admission
- planned, consistently implemented, evaluated individualised care
- documented problems reflecting the activities of living (AL)
- psychological factors need addressing
- goal-setting/outcomes need addressing

Feedback meeting

The findings were presented to the nursing staff of the three wards within the surgical unit, and a decision was made as to which ward would participate in the next phase of the study. The significance of this meeting cannot be overestimated. In some ways it was *the* most important meeting as the decision to formally undertake the study had to be agreed with the nurses (day and night staff) present including the nurse unit manager (NUM).

I arrived at the meeting with the triangulated findings (including table 4.7). I decided to also distribute copies of an article entitled 'Action Research' (Webb 1991) to reinforce information on the

Table 4.7: Congruent perceptions elicited from triangulation of data sources.

Congruent perceptions	Data sources
appropriate written assessment within 24 hours of admission	self-rating scale patient interviews patient care plans
planned, consistently implemented, evaluated, individualised care	self-rating scale patient interviews patient care plans
documented problems reflect the activities of living	self-rating scale patient care plans
psychological factors need to be addressed	self-rating scale patient interviews patient care plans
goal-setting/outcomes need to be addressed	self-rating scale patient care plans

research design and to emphasise the essential role of the ward staff in the study. The consent forms for staff were also needed.

I wanted the first meeting to be as informal and relaxed as possible, I took notes rather than used the micro-cassette. Individuals might have been intimidated by its presence and inhibited from participation.

The newly appointed NUM (we met for the first time at the meeting) was also present. The healthcare assistants and agency nurses staffed the ward for the hour to enable the qualified staff to attend. My strategy, after distributing drinks and biscuits, was to provide an introduction to action research emphasising the co-researcher role of the participants. No one had any knowledge of action research (which I had anticipated) or had even heard of the term. Some of the staff had facilitated reflective practice for student nurses, including the use of reflective journals but had never completed one themselves.

The findings from the patient interviews were presented. The categorisation process was explained, and an individual copy of all the findings was provided. I did not reveal the triangulated data until the staff had time to discuss what they believed were the most significant findings. The discussion centred around: astonishment at the fact that some patients thought that they needed permission to read their care plans and dismay that so many patients had turned to another health-care professional regarding their psychological needs. The physiotherapist is a valued and popular member of the ward team, and the nurses agreed that they felt she did appear to have more time than they did to spend with patients.

> Fiona: *Maybe it's to do with how she organises her time.*

There was surprise that discharge planning had not occurred for some of the patients; the positive comments regarding the bedside handover were rewarding; concern was expressed, however, regarding the fact that some patients felt inhibited/unable to comment on their care and that the references made to pain prevented independence.

A handout with the scoring systems for the self-rating scale and care plan evaluation tool together with details of the highest- and lowest-scoring items was distributed. In an attempt at avoiding the consequences of information overload, I explained how I had tried to compare the findings but emphasised that *they* would determine the focus for the study. The outcome of the meeting resulted in the decision to explore the problem of addressing patients' psychological needs while in hospital.

> Night sister: *Often we look at things from how we see them, especially psychological needs, not as the patient views them. I think we sometimes miss the vital bit.*

Selection of ward and co-researchers

I knew many of the nurses on B and C wards but had worked more with the staff of A ward. At the feedback meeting the staff on A ward seemed happy to 'give it a go', whereas on the other two wards there was noticeable reticence. The NUM supported this decision as the skill mix was relatively stable whereas B and C wards had fewer nurses at that time and currently more agency staff.

The ward that was utilised for the study had 22 beds. Patients undergoing breast, arterial and vein, gastric and bowel, gall bladder surgery and amputation of limbs were routinely cared for, as were patients with pancreatitis and chronic leg ulcers. The average throughput of patients per month was 120. Four surgeons admitted patients to the ward, which had three, six-bedded, bays and one of four beds. Both male and female patients were admitted for surgery but were nursed in separate bays.

I valued the working relationships that I had established with the sister of A ward and her team. We shared similar values regarding the standard of surgical care provision. Neither of us, fortunately, had developed the institutionalised approach to care, which can develop in the 'total institution' (Goffman 1961), as, when in an effort to bring order and control to the working day and 'get through the work', the nurse can inflict upon the patient a degree of order and control that denies the patient even the most basic of human rights, dignities and freedoms. This reinforces dependence (Wright 1989). I acted as action researcher/facilitator to the study; my peers, the ward staff, were the co-researchers.

The nursing philosophy of care on ward A equated with that of the RLT model of nursing. The model's concepts and assumptions provide the framework within which patient care is assessed, planned, implemented and evaluated. The system of ward organisation was 'team nursing'. There were two teams with six trained nurses in each, with two supporting healthcare assistants. Internal rotation could be negotiated to complement the permanent night staff. A night sister covered the surgical unit.

Ward staff act as clinical facilitators and assessors for student nurses on surgical placements. There was a large resources room for staff off the main corridor of the ward, which contained a computer, current nursing literature, visual displays of surgical operations and goals of nursing care, and medical equipment. The room was easily accessible from the ward. There was very little opportunity for privacy, and noise from the corridor was audible. All the meetings for this study were held there.

Staff capacity increased on ward A during the initial data collection phase (phase 1 of the study); so phase 2 commenced with 12 nurses on ward A, which included day and night sisters (table 4.8). To protect anonymity and confidentiality pseudonyms have been used. During the 15-month study, two of the staff nurses took up new posts, one abroad. They both left before the implementation of the change strategies. The two who replaced them appeared to very quickly identify with the team and contribute at the meetings. From their evaluation interviews, held at the close of the study, it was evident that initially they had had quite different perspectives:

> Geraldine: *I knew it had started because Sister told me at the interview. It was good to have the chance to learn all the new things that were going on. No, I didn't feel apprehensive; it was good to do something different.*
> Hannah: *When I knew of the project, I thought it would be one of those things that is done in theory but never*

Table 4.8: Clinical gradings of co-researchers on ward A.

Name	Grade
Day sister	G
Night sister	G
Lorraine (night duty)	E
Anne	F
Benita	D
Caroline	D
Denise	E
Fiona	E
Geraldine	D
Hannah	D
Esther	E
Jane	D

actually done in practice. Basically, I was for it; it sounded great in theory, but I thought we would meet up with nothing but problems.

Moving forward

Towards the end of the feedback meeting, the option of completing a short, anonymous questionnaire to gauge the nurses'/co-researchers' expectations of the study was provided and undertaken by all the ward A staff present. The questionnaire provided me with insights into how the co-researchers were feeling about their potential involvement in the study and about keeping a reflective journal (tables 4.9 & 4.10). I also needed to identify as early as possible any overt or potential resistance to change. I concluded by agreeing a strategy of weekly meetings to create a mutually supportive environment. These meetings would enable us to reflect on patient-centred problems, current nursing practices and plan strategies for change.

Co-researchers' final comments

Night sister: *The need for honest feelings if we are to gain from this.*
Day sister: *I hope we can keep it going and get the benefit for patients and all staff concerned.*
Esther: *Wish me luck!*

Table 4.9: Expectations of the study.

What are your expectations of the action research study?

I hope to learn from the experience and more about myself.

Gain further knowledge, increase my skills and learn from the group.

Become, hopefully, a more useful member of the ward team and enable us to become better nurses.

To gain knowledge and greater self-awareness, to improve as a nurse.

To learn and generate new ideas, to improve patient care. To learn more about myself and others.

Hopefully, I'll gain from it. I'll learn how to keep a reflective journal and better understanding of why I do what I do or why I shouldn't.

To improve my standard of care for the patients. Find out more about my good and my weak points.

I feel that perhaps this will help my patients and me: an improved way of looking at the care we all give.

Encourage to think more about why we do things and what effect that behaviour has on others, therefore help us to deal more effectively with patients' needs. I might learn to stop and think about things before doing them without thinking about the consequences.

I'm interested but a little nervous. I'll gain greater insight into myself.

To improve my knowledge of patients' needs and help me to understand what I and colleagues feel about situations.

Table 4.10: Nurses' feelings about keeping a reflective journal.

How do you feel about keeping a reflective journal?

A little anxious.

Okay. It will be difficult I think but useful for me.

Wondering if I'll find the time off duty. A little apprehensive.

Fine at present.

I don't mind; I'm just not sure what I'm supposed to be doing.

Mixed feelings - apprehension mainly.

Okay.

Keen but a little worried about it.

I feel it would enable me to think through all the procedures I do routinely and see how I feel about them and how they affect my patients and colleagues.

A little apprehensive of being open about my feelings.

Apprehensive and shy.

Chapter 5
The evolving action research process

'A precondition of action research is that participants perceive a need to initiate change and are willing to engage with research to scrutinise their work.' (Meyer 2001)

Structure of phase 2

Phase 2 of the study addresses the planning, implementation and evaluation of nurse-led change and development identified and undertaken by the co-researchers of ward A. The stages and methods used are summarised in table 5.1.

Table 5.1: The stages and methodology of the action research process and the resultant innovations.

STAGES	METHODS
PHASE 1 1. PROBLEM IDENTIFICATION	* Nurses' self-rating scale (22) * Patient interviews (8) * Nurses' care plan analysis (8)
PHASE 2 2. PLANNING	* Audiotaped group discussions/ focused reflections (16)

3. IMPLEMENTATION
   a) Patient self-medication
   b) Patient drug information leaflets
	* Collaborative approach
	* Protocol/leaflet writing
	* Audiotaped group analysis/
	   problem-solving

c) Patient-controlled analgesia	* Collaborative approach * Audiotaped group analysis/ problem-solving

(contd)

Table 5.1: (contd).

STAGES	METHODS
d) Operation-specific patient information leaflets	* Individual nurse ownership * Criteria for choice
4. EVALUATION a) Patient self-medication and drug information leaflets	* Patient pilot questionnaire (4) * Patient evaluation tool (17) * Multi-professional team evaluation tool (11)
b) Patient-controlled analgesia	* Patient evaluation tool (8) * Multi-professional team evaluation tool (14)
c) Operation-specific patient information leaflets	* Patient leaflet questionnaire
d) Action research study (15 months duration)	* Nurses' semi-structured interviews (12) * NUM unstructured interview

The process of change is documented from the description and analysis of the methods listed in table 5.1 and from my reflective notes. The concepts identified within critical social theory, reflective theory and change theory were in evidence particularly during this phase. Other concepts found relevant to the change process were also identified.

Ward A group meetings

Meetings with ward A staff (the co-researchers) were originally planned to be held in the ward seminar room from 2 p.m. to 3 p.m. once a week. We, the day staff and I, offered to rotate the times of the meetings to accommodate the night nurses, but this was declined. Consequently, they always attended in their off-duty time. This commitment was very evident amongst the day staff too; they often attended in their off-duty and during annual leave (sometimes with children in tow). For the staff who were unable to attend, I either ensured that other nurses provided their colleagues with the information and/or I wrote up the key points immediately following the meeting and forwarded the information in the internal post. However, on occasions co-researchers told me that they had not received information.

The nurse unit manager (NUM) had an open invitation to attend at any time. Yet she either gave advance notice to attend or 'dropped in' for the last fifteen minutes as she felt her presence could have intimidated some of the nurses, especially during the reflection sessions. She was kept up to date by either the ward sister or me. I forwarded every handout to her that I distributed to the co-researchers.

The meetings, although planned on a weekly basis, did not always take place. This was always due to the pressure of work. No patient could be put at risk by nurses attending the meetings; consequently, I had to cancel five meetings in all. Whenever possible, at the instigation of the NUM, nurses from the adjacent surgical wards or bank/agency nurses were brought in to cover; nevertheless, the cancelled meetings contributed to delayed decision-making and implementation of planned strategies. The initial feedback meeting (see pages 89–94) was held in November, and it was agreed to commence the study after Christmas, early in the new year.

The 16 meetings that were held were well attended, informal, enabled colleagues to wind down, socialise and digress, as well as address the fundamental aspects of the action research cycle. Initial suspicion of the micro-cassette referred to as 'that thing' was soon overcome. When confidential information about patients was discussed and derogatory remarks made about personnel, I was instructed to turn off the audiotape.

Once the innovations (see table 5.1, item 3 a-d) had been identified, the meetings addressed action planning, problem-solving and ongoing evaluations. All the initiatives were discussed at each meeting, but each is described and analysed independently in order to enable a clear explication of each innovation.

Preparing the co-researchers

The decision had been made to explore the psychological needs of surgical patients (see page 91). The next phase of the action research cycle was to facilitate reflection and discourse amongst the co-researchers. However, owing to the apprehensive feelings of eight of the nurses, as evidenced by their written comments (see tables 4.9 and 4.10) and verbal responses at the feedback meeting regarding keeping a reflective journal and sharing perspectives, I felt that there needed to be mutual recognition of current knowledge and clinical expertise as a way of initiating psychological safety. According to Minardi and Riley (1988), psychological safety centres around the ability to communicate to an individual that their beliefs, values, needs and wishes are recognised and understood in an open and non-judgmental way.

We each identified our position on 'the professional practice continuum' as described by Powell (1989) in her article 'The Reflective Practitioner in Nursing'. I also adapted an instrument for structured reflection originally devised and published by Johns (1993), to that of a focused reflection tool to accommodate the RLT model. By the second meeting I found that I had made an error of judgement, I had not consulted with my co-researchers regarding this tool, and they did not feel that it would facilitate the reflection process. They consequently devised a more appropriate tool to meet their needs (table 5.2).

Table 5.2: Co-researchers' tool for focused reflection.

For each meaningful/problematic event documented:

- Describe the event.
- What was I trying to achieve?
- What did the patient (others) feel?
- How did I feel?
- What were the consequences of my actions?
- On reflection, what would I do differently next time?

RLT model - How does this experience reflect:

- patient participation?
- patient independence?
- meeting psychological needs?
- the developmental stage of the patient?
- achievement of the activities of living?

Literature regarding surgical patients' anxieties/psychological stress was also discussed at the second meeting. Biley (1989) compares a convenience sample of 19 surgical nurses' and 20 pre-operative surgical patients' perceptions of potential stressors following surgery. Twenty-seven items, drawn from existing literature, were rank ordered by the two samples. Rank order correlation coefficient using Pearson's r showed a significant positive correlation between the scores on each question from all nursing staff and all patients ($r = + 0.69$, $p < 0.001$). 'Being in pain' was identified by patients as causing most worry; nurses ranked this item third.

Biley (1989) concludes that, as stress is so difficult to identify, even if a comprehensive assessment system is used, an effective approach may be to supply appropriate information and teach more general coping techniques. A holistic approach is required when providing information pre-operatively and caring for patients in pain due to the subjective nature of the experience. The co-researchers were familiar with earlier studies undertaken by Hayward (1975) and Boore (1978), which support the hypothesis that giving relevant information to patients pre-operatively would reduce post-operative pain. Teasdale (1993) in his critical appraisal of the hypothesis that information giving relieves anxiety, argues that this is an oversimplification. He concludes that one strategy for relieving patient anxiety is to adopt (further) empowering interventions. According to Phippen (1980), psychological stress can be increased by dependence (on nurses), which reduces an individual's self-esteem. As a result of this discussion the co-researchers decided to focus on the need to promote both physical and psychological independence in the relief of pain.

As the ward meetings evolved and innovations were identified, searching the literature and sharing knowledge and ideas became an ongoing process to determine current knowledge and strategies for change. Of necessity was the need to determine the co-researchers' teaching skills as patient-focused innovations would require patient education. Only the G grades had undertaken any formal teaching courses. However, the nurses were clinical facilitators for student nurses; so I tried to build on this knowledge and hoped that I did not appear to patronise them. A self-assessment tool (Bellman 1994, Spiers 2000, table 5.3) and patient teaching guidelines for the co-researchers were developed.

Table 5.3: Self-assessment for patient educators.

- How confident do I feel about teaching patients?
- Do I have the appropriate knowledge and skills?
- Am I familiar with contemporary issues in adult learning?
- How can I apply these to my patients?
- Which factors will promote a good learning environment for patients?
- Which factors may hinder patient teaching?
- What further knowledge and skills do I need to facilitate patient education?
- How will I gain these?

We started to explore the factors that promote a good learning environment for patients. For example:

> Loretta: *Well, these guidelines are meant to be helpful,*
> *but you can do what you like with them.* [laughter] *So*

> *let's now think about factors which promote a good*
> *learning environment.*
> Day sister: *Good interpersonal skills.*
> Benita: *Good knowledge-base.*
> Denise: *Encourage other patients to participate.*
> Day sister: *Yes; this is how you open the* [patient self-
> medication] *locker. Your tablets look good; here, have*
> *one of mine!* [much laughter]

Confidence building was much in evidence:

> Denise: *I don't feel very confident teaching patients.*
> Caroline: *We've got loads of reading to do.*
> Loretta: *I personally don't think so. I think you've got the*
> *knowledge; just think of the drugs in common use.*
> Day sister: *Yes, and you've got to be careful not to*
> *frighten them with too much information so they'll*
> *worry so much they won't take their medicines.*

Identifying the innovations

At only the third meeting, with nine of the co-researchers present, three innovations were identified, which were perceived as meeting patients' psychological needs, addressing the dependence-independence continuum of the RLT model, and as empowering for patients. These were patient self-medication (or self-administration of drugs), patient-controlled analgesia and operation-specific patient information leaflets as previously identified in table 5.1, items 3 a,c,d). It was certainly not my intention to undertake three innovations at any one time. The literature certainly advises against such folly as the chances of success are greatly reduced; yet there was much enthusiasm from the co-researchers for all of them. Two of the innovations, patient self-medication (PSM) and patient-controlled analgesia (PCA) would have to be undertaken in collaboration with members of the multi-professional team.

The decision to implement PSM evolved from the group reflecting on a specific incident described by day sister from her reflective journal. Owing to the demands of a busy surgical environment, she had (once again) been delayed in starting the drug round; consequently, many patients received their medications late, and she was constantly apologising for this. One patient, who was considered to be very demanding, became extremely aggressive.

Day sister: *I threw two lots of her pills away that day. She got me so confused I wasn't sure I'd given her the right ones. I feel anxiety was making her behave like this. She'd been here before, and, though in the past she wasn't a model patient, she is now going to lose both her legs. It's hard because of her very aggressive attitude, and I feel she mistrusts us. She resented giving us her pills on admission, complains that we never give them to her at the right time. She now feels I'm incapable of giving her pills.*

Hannah: *I felt sorry for her She was crying and obviously frustrated not being in charge of herself. I felt sorry for her not being in control.*

Day sister: *She told me she was the head of her family and had control of what went on. Yes, it must be very hard.*

Loretta: *What sort of solutions can you come up with, is there anything you can suggest about the drugs?*

Day sister: *Well, now we just show her every bottle. I suppose it would be better for her to do it herself, but we're not allowed to do it.*

Loretta: *What do you mean you're not allowed to do it?*

Day sister: *Well, there is self-medication, but I don't think pharmacy would allow us.*

Loretta: *Someone like her though, it would be quite appropriate?*

Day sister: *Yes, I'm sure it would.*

Loretta: *Well, I mean how do you feel about it generally?*

Day sister: *Self-medication. Sounds brilliant.*

Anne: *Well, patients often take their own tablets if the doctor hasn't come to write them up on admission.*

Patient-controlled analgesia (PCA) was raised by Denise. She had noted over the previous week (and since the second meeting and the discussion on psychological stress) the number of times she had been delayed in administering post-operative analgesia to her patients. She had worked in another unit where PCA had been unsuccessfully implemented but believed the strategy should again be attempted as it would address both psychological and physical patient independence. The NUM approved of the innovations. The timing was most significant.

She informed us that a consultant anaesthetist had also been considering PCA implementation.

The operation-specific information leaflets were not directly initiated via reflective practice. Some leaflets had previously been written, but problems had occurred regarding potential complexity of information for patients; none had been piloted on patients or read by colleagues. It was also agreed to value the work that had already started and include this strategy in the action research process.

As I concluded the meeting I decided (reflection in action) to ask each co-researcher individually to openly state their commitment to undertaking three key innovations together, as one innovation at any one time was deemed sufficient (see page 28). They each agreed and convinced me that the action plans that were to be devised would enable staggered implementation of the three initiatives. Well-motivated and intentioned as the group appeared to be, there were good-humoured reservations voiced: 'What have we let ourselves in for? Hope it won't be too much of a challenge!'

Factors related to group dynamics, social norms and the leadership influence of the G grades may have biased the decisions of some of the co-researchers. Yet all the co-reseachers present had voiced their opinions in a lively and open discussion.

The time scales for the implementation of the three innovations overlapped. PCA commenced in the middle of May for three months and became ongoing; PSM began the last week in August for a two-month trial period and subsequently also continued. The leaflets were completed and utilised throughout phase two.

Patient self-medication (PSM)

PSM was identified as an innovation, which, it was perceived, would promote the optimum level of patient independence and empower patients to participate in and have some control over their care. The traditional practice on the ward was for the nurse to remove a patient's medication on admission, lock it away and, when prescribed by the medical staff, administer it during drug rounds. This controlled method of drug administration disempowered patients and did not promote patient education about all aspects of their medication, check understanding or assess for potential problems.

> It seems contradictory to refuse patients the right to
> independent administration of medicines on admisssion
> [should their medical condition allow], yet expect them

> to regain independence the moment they are
> discharged from hospital. (Davis 1991, 29)

Action planning involved

- intra-professional and multi-professional working and user involvement - seeking the views of the patients, district and ward pharmacist, ward physiotherapist, nursing colleagues and consultants and junior medical staff
- reviewing written evidence - accessing, disseminating and critically analysing current literature on PSM amongst the co-researchers
- identifying resources and seeking information from two hospitals in the southeast - one was in the process of implementing and the other had implemented PSM
- devising a protocol

These processes resulted in shared co-researcher knowledge development, collaboration, individual and collective responsibility and feedback.

Patient self-medication literature

Despite published literature on PSM over the past twenty-five years, the concept has not been widely implemented (Davis 1991). Where it has been implemented, some areas provide a glowing account of the implementation process (Scriven 1987); other reports highlight the difficulties especially in relation to power and control by pharmacists (Baker and Pearson 1993). The collaborative approach to change used in this study enhances the partnership nature of the multi-professional healthcare team (Roper et al. 1990). Cottrell (1990) explains the pharmacist's role in careful planning and co-operative teamwork to successfully implement PSM, while the Guild of Hospital Pharmacists (1990) provide a memorandum of guidance.

There are potential problems with implementation. Not all patients will want to undertake PSM, they may wish to be exempted from social roles and responsibilities, adopting the 'sick role' (Parsons 1951). Not all nurses may advocate PSM, because they may not want to relinquish control over people's lives (Thompson et al. 1988), and may believe that it is quicker to do things themselves than educate and supervise patients (Gillis 1988). Patient non-comprehension may be the most common cause of non-compliance.

Advocates of PSM identify many positive patient outcomes. These include patient independence (Thomas 1992), and patient control and compliance (Scriven 1987). PSM enables patients to practise taking their drugs under supervision, alerts healthcare workers to any problems, provides an education programme and demonstrates trust - all of which have obvious psychological benefits for the patients and raise morale (Bird and Hassall 1993).

There are potential risks, however, and these have been identified as overdose, either intentional or accidental, under-dosage/forgetting to take the tablet, theft of a drug from another self-medicating patient and non-compliance. Bird and Hassall (1993) state that in five years of undertaking PSM they have experienced very few problems. Disadvantages of PSM are found to be few by Davis (1991), and no significant problems are identified by Scriven (1987). Verbal verification was provided by the sister of a surgical nursing development unit (NDU). Information was reviewed from two hospitals in the southeast, which were preparing to/had implemented PSM. The co-researchers carefully weighed up the pros and cons and decided that the benefits appeared to outweigh the possible risks, as reflected in extracts from their meetings:

Co-researchers' views of PSM

> Night sister: *Don't you think we are all so paranoid? We treat everybody the same, as if they're all going to steal drugs. If it goes towards empowering patients, we should try it and do it properly.*
> Ward pharmacist: *I'm all for it. We've all agreed it's a good idea, but how to go about it?*
> Day sister: *What if you have a patient who's a drug addict, and he sees all the other patients self-medicating?*
> Night sister: *Well, it might be good for him to do it, mightn't it? You're giving him the responsibility, trusting him and you're educating him at the same time.*
> Day sister: *What would happen if he stores up analgesia?*
> Caroline: *The patients should sign - will they be accountable?*
> Ward pharmacist: *We'll have to explore all that.*

Seeking patients' views on the need for PSM

To gauge the need for and the potential success of the initiative anecdotal information was fed back to the meetings:

> Lorraine: *It was embarrassing, as I gave Mr G. his night sedation I said: 'Now don't leave them on your locker; remember to take them.' He said: 'I never forget. I've been taking them for years.'*
> Geraldine: *I asked Mrs F. She said that she'd be quite happy to do her own tablets. She then produced a detailed list of her drugs with the times she took them and then half an hour later asked me when she could start taking her own tablets!* [laughter]

What was so enlightening and surprising for all the co-researchers was the large number of patients who had no idea why they were prescribed medication. Many also had little or no knowledge of the side effects of the drugs they were taking.

> Day sister: *When I asked Mrs S. if she knew what her tablets were for she said: 'I've been taking them for ten years because the doctor told me to, but I don't know what they're for.'*
> Jane: *Patients often don't know what their drugs are for. When I asked one patient the other day, she said no one had ever asked her that question before. Then, after thinking for a moment, she said: 'Why should I take these tablets if I don't know what they're for?'*

Devising PSM protocol

The co-researchers, by anonymous ballot, identified four colleagues to write up the protocol: day sister, Anne (F grade), Fiona (E grade) and the night staff nurse (E grade) Lorraine. Taking time out to think and write was crucial to the success of the study and especially so on this occasion to enable the production of a draft protocol. Sister, Anne and Fiona (Lorraine, the night nurse was in the end unable to attend) eventually met to produce the document, which they completed during one span of duty, in the seminar room. The NUM guaranteed that cover was provided for the ward. Feedback from colleagues was very positive.

> Loretta: *The protocol is looking good. I'm very impressed. How do you feel about us making some comments?*
> Day sister: *Fine, we expect it to be pulled apart, because we have never done it before.*

> Night sister: *You did it so fast. I'm sure some people would spend a couple of months on this, well done.*
> Day sister: *Well, we started at 10 and finished at 3.30. Hannah typed it up for us.*
> Fiona: *I must admit we did a lot of reading and pinched stuff.*
> Loretta: *But that's shared knowledge, which serves to benefit patients.*
> Ward pharmacist: *This is very good. The only other protocol I've seen was from E ward, and it was dreadful. There was nothing in it.*
> Day sister: *I know, they're still using the drug trolley.*
> Denise: *They're playing at it.*
> Night sister: *Either do it or don't do it - don't pretend. Now, could we just change this word here 'hindered' maybe to 'compromised'? Now, it's up to you.*
> Day sister: *No, it isn't. It's up to everyone.*

The people to whom draft copies of the protocol were to be sent were agreed by the co-researchers. It was sent for comment to all the co-researchers (as only three had originally devised it), the NUM, the district pharmacist, the ward pharmacist, the legal department, nurses on the adjoining surgical wards, the ward physiotherapist, the stomatherapist and myself. There was a difference of opinion, however, regarding the consultants (see below).

Day sister met with the district pharmacist.

> Day sister: *Provided we put the bits in that pharmacy wanted, she couldn't see that there was going to be any problem.*
> Loretta: *I'm just so surprised that she approved it without any hassle! It's just incredible!*

Since the commencement of phase two of the study, I had been trying to identify the resisters to change. There was no overt resistance from any of the co-researchers or, as far as I could tell, from any directly associated personnel. However a pharmacist from an adjoining ward had been making negative comments about self-medication and the information produced for patients:

> Fiona: *She was very anti. I think it was sour grapes.*

The NUM sought advice from the legal department. Only minor rewording to the protocol was required.

PSM and the medical staff

The NUM and day sister offered to sound out the consultants. They all approved, including the consultant who was originally opposed to the study (page 70). One of the consultants, Mr Y., was the chair of the Drug and Therapeutics Committee, which would eventually have to approve the protocol and sanction the initiative.

> Day sister: *Quite honestly, I don't think it's worth giving a copy* [of the protocol] *to the consultants as they'll just put it in the bin.*
> Loretta: *Although, Mr Y. will eventually get one as he's the chair of the Drug committee.*
> Day sister: *Oh, yes, but he'll pull it apart.*
> Loretta: *But it might be useful for him to pull it apart, as we have a couple of weeks to play with before the next committee meets.*

A general discussion ensued. I was faced with a dilemma. I felt that although the consultants had agreed in principle, we all knew, although it was never voiced, that such is their power, that any one of them could have stalled or even halted the process. The co-researchers, although having written and approved the protocol, were still aware of this potentially restraining force.

> Loretta: *Going back to the consultants. Maybe Mr Y. to start with and then, once he has made comments, send it out to the others. You could ask them for comments, but you don't have to follow them.* [laughter]

At the following meeting sister produced a very supportive letter from Mr Y. complimenting the staff on their achievement to date (box 5.1). In spite of this response nurse-doctor communications remained a controversial issue. At one meeting the co-researchers discussed the implications of PSM for the medical staff.

> Geraldine: *The doctors will need re-educating as they will have to write everything as TTOs.* [laughter]

Loretta: *So who's going to deal with the doctors?*
Day sister: *Don't all look at me like that!* [laughter]
Jane: *Well, what's going to be different for them?*
Esther: *Well, they are going to have to prescribe on a different part of the drug chart.*
Benita: *And they are going to have to look at the prescriptions more often.*
Anne: *And it's going to have to be written much clearer for the patients to read.*

Box 5.1: Letter of support from a consultant surgeon.

Dear Sister,

Proposal for self-medication

This looks absolutely great and I am 100% behind you. I would actually like to introduce it universally throughout the Unit, rather than wait for the pilot studies, but it may be that we will have to persuade a few people before the introduction.

If there is any way in which I can help, other than through the Drug and Therapeutics Committee, please let me know.

You are quite right that as medical and nursing staff we owe our patients a duty of care, and a pre-requisite of allowing self-medication is a formal assessment and record showing that the patient is competent and capable of managing the procedure.

In the ward environment, it is certainly possible that other patients or visitors can have access to such drugs, and, if loss or damage occurs as a result, the Authority would be legally liable. In order to minimise this risk, patients who are allowed to administer their own drugs must be provided with a locked drawer or cupboard in which the medicines can be kept and the patient made responsible for the custody and safe-keeping of the key.

Yours sincerely,

Chairman
Drug and Therapeutics Committee

PSM resources

While the protocol was being discussed, night sister identified the need to complement verbal drug information with written drug information leaflets. This strategy for reinforcement was also perceived as time-saving for the nurse. A democratic approach to devising them was adopted; each co-researcher identified one or two drugs in common use. Once written, the leaflets were subjected to group scrutiny and were sent to the ward pharmacist for comment. This became an ongoing process.

Individual-locking bedside medicine cabinets were chosen from a catalogue and a key board ordered. The NUM priced the cabinets and arranged for a representative to demonstrate them to the co-researchers on the ward. The ward pharmacist arranged the production of self-medication stickers. Underlying anxieties emerged in the form of humour and laughter as the proposed innovation became a reality.

> Day sister: *As the patients arrive, we'll assess them. Pharmacy have supplied the stickers.*
>
> Lorraine: *Where will we stick them?*
>
> Fiona: *On their drug chart, on their bed, on their forehead - they'll be everywhere!*
>
> Loretta: *Yes, then there's the key. Where are they going to keep their key?*
>
> Day sister: *Put them on a chain around their neck! No. I've ordered a key board as a central point for them. You'll be able to check at a glance which patients have their own key. Then there's numbering them, labelling them and if they get mislaid ... We'll be tearing our hair out - can we change our minds!*

Implementing PSM

The Drug and Therapeutics Committee approved the protocol and advocated a two-month pilot study. To the co-researchers this appeared to be rather a short time span in which to evaluate a major innovation especially as the number of patients self-medicating at any one time would fluctuate significantly.

Implementation was delayed by seven weeks, however, for two reasons. The locking cabinets had to be hand-made, and there was slippage on the delivery date. Far more overwhelming was a situation that had never previously occurred to any of the co-researchers before but which left us all devastated and seriously considering abandoning the innovation. A female patient, with a history of mental illness, was admitted for surgery. She did not hand over her drugs on admission but said that her family would bring them in later that day. Unknown to the nurses she had hidden them in her bedside locker. She took an overdose that evening and was found dead early the next morning.

Profound feelings of distress were felt by all the staff. Group meetings continued where mutual support and open discussion were encouraged. The co-researchers eventually decided to proceed with PSM. They reasoned that this had been an extremely rare occurrence, that they would be acutely aware of the possibility in the future, that they had invested a great deal of themselves and hospital monies in the project to date and that the outcome would benefit many surgical patients.

The delay to the implementation date meant that day sister was on annual leave when PSM commenced. However, her co-researchers felt reasonably confident that they could initiate the process. At the meeting immediately preceding the start date they displayed positive attitudes and elation and, understandably, anxieties related to the risk taking of any new strategy:

> Anne: *It's difficult to imagine as none of us have had this experience before. We're all just learning. We'll have to deal with each issue as it comes.*

On admission the nurse assessed each patient's suitability for PSM from identified criteria. If the patient wished to be self-medicating, they then signed the form to accept responsibility for storing, administering and recording their medication and for the safe custody of the cabinet key. The main problems initially were identified as being sure that the right decision was made as to a patient's suitability for PSM, four mislaid keys, some medical staff not being informed as to changes in writing up medications for PSM and difficulties with patients who were self-medicating being prescribed a new drug at the week-end. The group meetings, however, revealed the co-researchers' enthusiasm:

> Loretta: *How's self-medication going then?*
> Fiona: *Oh I've had loads and loads of patients doing it. Mrs S. is, so is Mrs T., and Mrs D. is about to.*
> Caroline: *Mrs S. said how confusing it was.*
> Fiona:"*Oh yes, it was just filling in the drug chart was too much for her. The others are taking it themselves lovely. Who else? Now, Mr B. he was, but he's gone home now.*
> Caroline: *Yes, he did very well.*
> Geraldine: *He was quite impressed by it.*

Evaluation of PSM

A strategy for evaluation was agreed. We devised a patient question-naire based on the literature and patients' and co-researchers' initial perceptions. The co-researchers agreed that I should pilot this tool on four patients, and some amendments to question structure were made accordingly. I sat with each patient as they completed the evaluation forms (table 5.4). Most significant was their delight at retaining control over their drugs, and three of the patients said that it showed that the nurses trusted them (which aids the patients' psychological needs). When the co-researchers remembered, patients who were self-medicating were then asked if they would like to complete the evaluation form prior to discharge. There were seventeen completed forms (table 5.1, item 4a, p. 96).

Table 5.4: PSM patient evaluation form.

Dear Patient,

Would you please give your views about the new medicine scheme on this ward? **We would appreciate your honest opinion**. There are no right or wrong answers. The forms are anonymous. Thank you for your help.

1. How do you feel about being responsible for your own medicines while in hospital?
2. Why do you think self-medication has been introduced in hospital?
3. What problems occurred when using the locking medicine cabinet?
4. Do you always take your own medicine or does the nurse or pharmacist assist you?
5. Have you had any problems e.g. ever fogotten to take any of your medicines, difficulty filling in the medicine chart?
6. Why did the doctor prescribe your medicine?
7. What information have you been given about your medicines? Did you find this information helpful?
8. When leaving hospital what might prevent you from continuing to take your medicine?
9. Is there anything else you would like to say about self-medication?

The discussions within the group meetings and the literature provided the questionnaire format that was devised for the multi-professional team. The co-researchers were asked to comment on the validity of the questions (table 5.5). Fiona offered to complete the form to provide constructive criticism on the design and format and to determine the approximate length of time required for completion. It was agreed that, as well as the co-researchers completing the form at the end of the two-month trial, three house officers and the physiotherapist would also be asked for their perceptions. However, the only received completed forms were from eleven co-researchers.

Table 5.5: Staff PSM evaluation form.

Please complete this form at your earliest convenience. There are no right or wrong answers, just personal reflections of the two-month pilot study.

1. How do you feel about patients being responsible for their own medication?
2. What are the advantages of this innovation:

   - for patients?
   - for you?
   - for the organisation?

3. What are the disadvantages of this innovation:

   - for patients?
   - for you
   - for the organisation?

4. If problems were experienced with the following, how were they resolved?

   - locking medicine cabinets
   - prescription charts
   - patient education
   - non-compliance
   - other

5. What do you like most about PSM? What do you like least about PSM?
6. Are there any other comments you would like to make regarding PSM?

Thank you for completing the evaluation form

All eleven co-researchers demonstrated positive feelings towards patients being responsible for their own medication. Overall it was viewed as a very good innovation. The advantages and disadvantages as perceived by the co-researchers are listed in tables 5.6 and 5.7 below. Their descriptions of what they liked most and least are in table 5.8

Table 5.6: Co-researchers' perceptions of the advantages of PSM for the patient, nurse and the organisation.

Advantages - patients	Advantages - nurses	Advantage - organisation
promotes independence	enhanced drug knowledge	potential cost saving
knowledge drugs/ side effects	potentially time saving	reduces drug errors
informed choice	smaller drug round	proactive, innovative clinical setting
optimum administration time	greater job satisfaction	up-to-date knowledgeable workers
patients believe they are helping the nurses	reduced workload	improves the quality of care
promotes compliance on discharge	nurse-patient communication improved	potential for reduced re-admission due to patient compliance
	improved teaching skills	

Table 5.7: Co-researchers' perceived disadvantages of PSM for patients, nurses and the organisation.

Disadvantages - patients	Disadvantages - nurses	Disadvantages - organisation
may feel less cared for	initially time consuming	potential risk of litigation
difficulty completing drug cards	increased paperwork	expense of setting up the scheme
physical difficulties	unsure when to restock drugs	provision of time to set up and implement PSM
potential information overload	difficulty remembering to give patients evaluation tool	provision of time for nurses to update their knowledge
forgetting to take medication	reduced contact with patients for some team members	increased workload for pharmacy

below. It was felt that more patients needed to be encouraged to self-medicate. Specific responses included:

- PSM gives patients a sense of being in control.
- PSM helps patients to understand their medication and side effects.
- PSM is the preferable way for drugs to be administered.
- Many patients are no less capable when in hospital.

Problems of implementing PSM were associated with:

- the locking medicine cabinets - nine co-researchers experienced no problems; however, one co-researcher had witnessed the difficulty of a patient in trying to reach the cabinet when confined to bed. Another co-researcher had to keep reminding a patient to keep his cabinet locked.
- prescription charts - eight co-researchers had to mark patients' charts for them. Of these patients, five had difficulty signing and three forgot to sign the chart.
- patient education - two co-researchers had to reinforce information verbally and re-explain the drug information leaflet. One co-researcher stated that some patients were not keen on being educated about their medication, 'ignorance is bliss'.

Table 5.8: Co-researchers' descriptions of what they liked most and least about PSM.

Liked most about PSM	Liked least about PSM
patients' involvement	increased accountability and responsibility
patients being in control helped to reduce their anxiety	reduced quality of information to patients when ward is busy
patients' independence enhanced	uncertainty of final outcome
patients able to initiate pain relief quickly	having to trust patients to take their own medication correctly
patients and nurses working together	'Trying to explain to a patient who, up until admission, was taking their own tablets that now I didn't think they could manage.'
ensures nurses stay up to date with drugs	'Potential for disaster!'
time saving	
potential for earlier discharge home	

- non-compliance - PSM had to be discontinued for one patient. One co-researcher stated that finding time for discussion, answering patients' questions, and getting feedback promoted compliance.

Patients' evaluation of PSM

All 17 patients who completed the self-medication questionnaire (table 5.4) were of British nationality. There were 13 female and four male patients (table 5.9).

Table 5.9: Patients who completed a self-evaluation questionnaire.

Age range	59–65	66–70	71–75	76–80	81–85	86–90
Female	3	5	3	1	–	1
Male	1	1	2	–	–	–
Total	4	6	5	1	–	1

All 17 patients responded positively to being responsible for their own medication while in hospital. PSM was thought to be a good idea for anyone capable of doing so. One patient said that you had to be responsible at home and another that if things go wrong it's your own fault. Table 5.10 demonstrates patients' responses to the question: Why do you think self-medication has been introduced in this ward?

Table 5.10: Patients' perceptions of reasons for PSM implementation.

Saves the nurses time (11)
Eases the nurses' workload (11)
Helps patients become knowledgeable about their medication (2)
Gets patients used to self-medicating for when they go home (2)
Makes patients more responsible (2)
Alleviates patients' fears that staff may fail in some way to continue treatment taken at home (1)
Cost saving (1)
Makes patients more aware of their condition (1)
Don't know (2)

Only one specific problem was identified with PSM. One patient who had difficulty sitting up in bed said that he could not always operate the key.

The information given to patients by the co-researchers included the action of each prescribed drug, the side effects of the drugs and reinforcement of information originally provided by the doctor and the pharmacist. Three patients received no information about their medications, but it may be that no further information was needed after a co-researcher's initial assessment. The information provided was found to be helpful by nine of the patients, some information was helpful according to two patients, and one did not feel it was helpful.

Patients were asked whether they understood why they were prescribed medication; their responses included:

- long-term medication - diabetes mellitus, high blood pressure, cardiac disease
- for pain
- for infection
- because I needed it
- iron for my blood
- to help me sleep
- for the operation
- don't know

Did patients want to know which side effects to look out for? Thirteen said that they did, and the same number knew which side effects to look out for. Nothing would prevent 14 of the patients from continuing to take medication on discharge. One said: 'Been taking them so long, I won't forget!'

Patients' additional comments
- Very good idea.
- I found it no problem at all.
- A very good idea if patient is willing.
- Good idea - gives people the opportunity to assist in their own recovery.
- Made me feel less dependent on the nurses.
- I was sure of getting all the tablets I needed to take.
- You know you are getting the right ones.

The patients did not experience any difficulty completing the questionnaires, and they provided the co-researchers with instant feedback.

The outcome of PSM

Advantages

All patients and staff responded positively to the use of PSM on the ward. The majority of patients felt that they were helping the nurses by self-medicating, whereas the co-researchers viewed PSM as a strategy for promoting independence and enhancing knowledge of drugs. Only one co-researcher felt that it reduced her workload; seven stated that PSM was more time-consuming. This is to be anticipated initially with any innovation that significantly changes practice.

Disadvantages

Very few disadvantages for patients were identified by the co-researchers; all the patients said that they had no problems with PSM. Eight co-researchers did identify drug-chart problems particularly in relation to patient difficulty with signing the chart and patients forgetting to sign. (This however was not the case for the seventeen patients who completed the evaluation questionnaire.) On reviewing the protocol, it was found that there was a discrepancy between instructions to patients to sign their drug chart and in the overall objectives, which refer to patients just ticking when they have taken the drug. This required clarification. However, it may be that patients can do neither yet are still able to administer and understand their drugs, as, for example, the partially sighted patient taking medication prior to hospitalisation.

Explanation of patient-specific problems

These may not be teething problems. The mean age of the sample was seventy years. With an increasingly older adult occupancy, the older surgical patient may need to have a chart designed specifically for their needs. This may mean a review of the current drug chart throughout the health district, especially when other areas implement PSM. Nurses signing the drug chart on behalf of patients partially negates the participatory nature of PSM (but still leaves the patient in control).

Advantages for the organisation

The co-researchers identified more advantages for the organisation than disadvantages. They focused on cost-effectiveness and a motivated workforce responding positively to change. There would be a potential reduction in drug errors and an increase in patient compliance. These positive outcomes are cited by Cottrell (1990), who also identifies a reduced rate of readmission. Bird and Hassall (1993) state that patient self-administration of drugs is more cost-effective and more satisfactory than readmission to hospital.

Outcome

I compiled a short report of the process and outcome of PSM and distributed it to the co-researchers and NUM. Copies were also sent to the chair of the Drug and Therapeutics Committee, the district pharmacist and the director of quality assurance (nursing). The group meetings continued to monitor the progress of this innovation (and the two others) and to further develop the co-researchers' knowledge and skills. A new drug chart is now being devised and the ward will be used as a resource for clinical areas now planning to implement PCA. Final interviews with the co-researchers were undertaken (as I withdrew from the project) three months after the implementation of PSM:

Co-researchers' views

> Fiona: *The innovation I think that gave me the most satis-faction was self-medication because it was actually something totally and utterly new. Most of the patients seemed really pleased with it. Most of them seemed quite chuffed that they could do it themselves. I liked that.*
>
> Day sister: *There were so many difficulties presented to us that I often thought: 'Are we ever going to get this?' But we actually worked them through ... and we did get it in the end; so I think this was quite an achievement, but sometimes I thought: 'Oh God, is it ever going to happen?' But it did. I quite enjoyed being involved in writing the protocol. It makes the patients more independent and more in control of what is going on rather than just keep shovelling tablets down them. It has definitely made a lot of them more questioning about what the tablets are for and why they are taking them and should they take this one with that one so I mean it has been very good for the patients.*
>
> NUM: *I am very pleased about the self-medication. Watching the patients self-medicate - they seem more at ease, more comfortable, talking to them they love it, it is good ... and the rest of the hospital will be very interested in what has been happening on self-medica-tion on the ward now that it is up and running.*

Patient-controlled analgesia

Patient-controlled analgesia (PCA) was introduced as the second innova-tion by the co-researchers to address the individualistic nature of post-operative pain, to facilitate psychological and physical independence and to empower patients - giving them control over their pain. Theatre nurses and members of the multi-professional team were also involved in the initiative, which included anaesthetists, consultants, house officers, pharmacists and the ward physiotherapist. The group meetings once again involved exploring the literature, sharing knowledge, planning a strategy and a time-scale for implementation.

An overview of the costs and benefits of PCA is provided by Thomas and Rose (1993), who assert that its efficacy in controlling pain and its popularity with patients and staff have ensured a wide clinical utility - PCA can reduce the length of hospital stay, save nurses time and therefore represents a cost-effective device. Side effects of nausea and vomiting produced by the opioids may modify analgesic consumption (Owen et al. 1988) and respiratory depression is a frequently voiced concern (Thomas and Rose 1993). This fear, however, is unfounded according to Bennett et al. (1982), who found no evidence of respiratory depression in 1300 patients.

A consultant anaesthetist had also been considering introducing PCA, and a meeting was held to discuss the initiative and review a PCA wristwatch infusor. This equipment appeared to be considerably more practical and user-friendly than the pump mechanism, which was cumbersome for patients attempting to mobilise post-operatively. The NUM arranged a ward-based demonstration by the company representative.

The equipment was to be stored and prepared in the pharmacy and sent to the operating theatre to be set up by an anaesthetist. The co-researchers, by using their professional judgement, were to assess each patient on admission as suitable for PCA and prepare them accordingly. Each selected patient also received a detailed explanatory leaflet provided by the manufacturers. There was a need to devise a protocol. However, it was first agreed to implement PCA for a three-month period, and evaluate the outcome from both the patients' and the multi-professional team's perspectives. The NUM, though, offered to write an initial draft protocol (for us all to review) but approximately one month into the project stated: 'I have written one, but I'm going to change it in light of the problems that have come up.'

Initial problems with PCA

The most significant problem appeared to be that, although patients were being prepared for PCA by the ward nurses, two of the anaesthetists were not commencing it in theatres:

> Day sister: *I saw Dr V.* [consultant anaesthetist]
> *yesterday, and she said that she must do something*

> about it. It's Dr M. we have to get organised to do it.
>
> Anne: *Every time we tell the patients they are going to get it, they don't get it.*
>
> Loretta: *I mean, it's daft really, isn't it? The equipment is just there.*
>
> Day sister: *But I knew this would happen as soon as it goes out of our hands and out of the ward and goes downstairs* [to recovery].
>
> Geraldine: *Well, I bet the nurses down there aren't pushing it, because it's more work.*
>
> Fiona: *They* [recovery nurses] *have to get them* [the anaesthetists] *to give a stat loading dose. There was one woman I nursed who wasn't given the loading dose* [in theatre]*; she was in agony poor thing. I had to get someone to give her a stat dose.*

It was agreed that sister and I would reinforce the process with the anaesthetists and recovery nurses:

> Day sister: *Dr E. was okay. He said we're supposed to be in the twenty-first century but some people are still living in the Dark Ages!*

Planned evaluation of PCA

The evaluation strategy was agreed by both the co-researchers and the consultant anaesthetist. It consisted of a form (collaboratively devised by myself, the consultant anaesthetist and the co-researchers) to be completed by an anaesthetist and ward nurse, which included details of PCA commencement and completion times, pain assessment chart details, the overall amount of drug utilised and the amount discarded. The literature provided previously validated questionnaires for both patients and the multi-professional team (Thomas 1993).

After a three-month trial period patients' and staff's perceptions of PCA were evaluated. Overall they were very favourable. There were still a number of problems to be addressed in spite of positive feedback from one of the ward consultants.

> NUM: *He said he thought it was the best thing since sliced bread and all his patients are going to have it.*

The co-researchers and consultant anaesthetist agreed that 20 patients were to be asked by the co-researchers whether they would complete an evaluation questionnaire. Only eight were completed.

The lack of completed questionnaires reflects three specific problems:

- patients who were given forms took them home with them to complete yet failed to return them;
- some patients were in possession of a form and were prepared for PCA yet failed to receive it;
- the co-researcher forgot to give the PCA patient an evaluation form.

A descriptive analysis of the qualitative data from the questionnaires was undertaken. In spite of the small response, some useful information was obtained that complemented the findings both from the literature and from the multi-professional team evaluation.

Multi-professional team's and patients' evaluation of PCA

The response rate for questionnaire completion is detailed in table 5.11

Table 5.11: Questionnaire response - multi-professional team.

Team members	No. sent	No. returned
Nurses	13	11
Anaesthetists	4	1
Medical staff	2	1
Physiotherapist	1	1
Total	20	14

The most important question was the extent to which PCA provided post-operative pain relief shown in table 5.12.

Table 5.12: Perceptions of PCA's efficacy.

How much pain relief do you think PCA provides?	Patients' response (eight respondents)	Team perceptions (14 respondents)
Relief most of the time	5	11
Relief a lot of the time	1	3
Relief some of the time	2	–
Relief very seldom	–	–

Of the five patients who had previously received other types of pain control three believed that PCA was much better and two better in comparison. The multi-professional team also felt that PCA was better (eight responses) and much better (six responses) than the intra-muscular method of pain relief. The patients' and team's most and least favourable perceptions of PCA are recorded in tables 5.13 and 5.14.

Table 5.13: Patients' most and least favoured perceptions of PCA.

Patients liked most about PCA	Patients liked least about PCA
Personal control (5)	A feeling of drowsiness (1)
Only used when needed (3)	Felt nauseated (1)

Table 5.14: Multi-professional team's perceptions of most and least favourable aspects of PCA.

Team liked most about PCA (14 respondents)	Team liked least about PCA
Patients are in control (11)	Some anaesthetists were not giving prepared patients the loading dose (10)
Patients did not have to ask for analgesia (4)	Patients who were prepared on the ward failed to receive PCA in spite of notifying theatres (4)
Patients did not have to wait to receive analgesia (4)	Delay for a patient due to waiting for cannula to be resited when it tissued (1)
Patients received a measured dose when they wanted it (3)	Difficulty in assessing the amount of analgesia received (1)
Immediate pain relief (5)	Unable to administer an anti-emetic by the same route (1)
No painful injections are required (5)	No way of telling if 'machine' is working (1)
Anxiety levels are reduced (2)	Uncertainty regarding method of disposal (2)
Patients mobilise more quickly (4)	Uncertainty regarding storing of PCA diffusors (1)
Saved the nurses time (6) (2 of the respondents were non-nurses)	

The most significant problems were the anaesthetists not providing a loading dose of the drug, which negates the effect of PCA, and the failure in the recovery ward to commence PCA for prepared patients. General perceptions of PCA were most favourable, table 5.15.

Table 5.15: Patients' and multi-professional team's feelings about PCA.

Patients (eight respondents)	Team (14 respondents)
I felt good being in control of my pain relief (3)	Very happy, totally in favour (9)
It gave me a feeling of security (1)	Excellent, provided patients fully understand (5)
Most satisfactory (1)	Better than nurses' subjective judgements about pain relief (3)
Quick and easy pain control when you need it (1)	Enhances patient independence (2)
I found all aspects very good, great to be in control of your pain (1)	Alleviates anxiety (2)
I was worried about the small amount of drug left when almost empty (1)	Patients are happier with it (2)
The rapid use of the drug worried me (1)	Provides participation in care (1)
Because it was explained to me properly, I understood it and it was a great help (1)	I am pleased to be involved in this innovation (1)

Multi-professional team's recommendations

The team's recommendations included exploring the extent of anti-emetic use with PCA, considering an alternative analgesia to reduce the effects of nausea in some patients and devising a protocol in collaboration with the anaesthetic and theatre staff. A report of the PCA process and outcomes was compiled and distributed to the co-researchers and the NUM. Copies were sent to the director of quality (nursing), the consultant anaesthetist, the district pharmacist and to the senior nurse manager (theatres).

Co-researchers' feedback

The final interviews that were undertaken with the co-researchers as I withdrew from the study (seven months after the implementation of PCA) revealed much enthusiasm for this initiative:

> Hannah: *I really liked* [implementing] *PCA. The patients think it's great.*

> Caroline: *PCA is simple to take on board. I remember thinking this is lovely, I'm really going to enjoy doing this and I did!*
>
> Esther: *It's excellent, the patients are so much better afterwards. You haven't got to keep stabbing them with needles, and their pain is relieved all the time, not just every four hours when you give them a booster. They mobilise quicker and recover a lot better.*
>
> NUM: *I must admit I think PCA has been the most beneficial of the innovations. It has now spread not only through the whole of the surgical unit it has now hit X hospital and Y hospital* [in the same health district] *The patients seem more independent, and they seem, when you go right up to them, far more relaxed and that, to me, to get on top of pain control post-operatively, is quite important. Nice to see that.*

Yet there were still problems:

> Benita: *PCA is still not being done effectively. We had a gentleman the other day, a young man in his late 30s for bowel surgery. He was very frightened. I didn't know whether to assess him or not in case it didn't happen. We did assess him, but then it ran out during the night and he was in agony. We must remember to keep checking it. In the end, the nurses took it out and gave him injections.*
>
> Day sister: *PCA has given me the least satisfaction, because it has been so difficult to get the initiative set up. Once it is up, it is so effective but it is actually getting it. You get so disappointed because you talk to the patients about it, you show them it, you write they are suitable and yet they still come back without it. I think, though, it is probably slowly getting better, but perhaps we expected too much too soon.*

Operation-specific information leaflets

The co-researchers each agreed to devise and pilot a specific leaflet. The assumption was that, by educating patients about their condition and the operation, they would feel less anxious and be more in control of their situation. The leaflets that had previously been devised (prior to the study) but not reviewed by the group or piloted were also included as there had been problems determining their level of complexity and use of medical terminology for patients:

> Day sister: *It was the technical bit about the op. I thought the patient would look at it and think, oh, what are they talking about? Difficult to know really.*

Previously devised leaflets included mastectomy, laporoscopic cholecystectomy, cholecystectomy, gastrectomy and diverticular disease. The co-researchers addressed this third initiative at the (previously discussed) planning meetings. Further leaflets were devised - small bowel surgery, large bowel surgery, thyroidectomy, pilonidal sinus and arterial surgery. Benita offered to co-ordinate the strategy as the initiative had originally been her idea.

Literature regarding writing and evaluating patient education leaflets was at that time virtually nonexistent. Taylor et al. (1982) pose the question - do patients understand patient-education brochures? The Health Education Council, which distributes millions of health information leaflets, was unable to assist; an officer stated that she knew at that time of no evaluation strategy that was in place. Ewles and Simnett (1992, 1999), however, give a 'criteria for choice', which provides prompts for leaflet production. They also cite the 'frequency of gobbledegook' formula, devised by Gunning (1968 in Ewles and Simnet 1992, 1999), which the co-researchers utilised to determine their leaflets' level of plain English and readability.

Evaluating information leaflets

An evaluation tool was devised by the co-researchers (see table 5.16).

> Loretta: *Okay so give me your ideas.*
> Fiona: *Did you find the leaflet helpful?*
> Lorraine: *Could you understand it?*
> NUM: *A brief sentence maybe saying exactly what they had done, in their own words.*
> Hannah: *Was there anything missing?*
>
> Day sister: *We don't want to make it too long do we or else they might get fed up? We could put do you feel you have enough information for when you go home?*
> Fiona: *No and they're still here 3 months later!* (much laughter)

> Day sister: *Now a problem if they don't speak English.*
> *What are we going to do?*
> NUM: *They can be sent to be translated, especially for*
> *our local Asian community.*
> Esther: *Maybe we should make a video!* (laughter)
> Loretta: *Fine so I'll get the form typed up to review at*
> *the next meeting.*

At the next meeting the patient evaluation form (table 5.16) was approved. Discussion followed as to whether to seek the views of the consultants regarding the leaflets and the evaluation tool. Anne offered to send the evaluation form and copies of each completed leaflet, but at the following meeting:

> Loretta: *So you were going to send them to the consul-*
> *tants to look at.*

Table 5.16: Patient leaflet evaluation questionnaire.

PATIENT LEAFLET QUESTIONNAIRE

Title of leaflet ....

Completing this form will help the nurses to review the information contained in the leaflet. There are no right or wrong answers, and the information is anonymous. Thank you for your help.

1. Did you find the leaflet helpful?
2. Was there enough information for you?
3. Was it easy to read?
4. Were the messages clear?
5. Were the explanations adequate?
6. Did the information help to reassure you?
7. Did any of the information worry you? If YES, what in particular?
8. Do you understand the reason for your operation?
9. Should any of the information in the leaflet be dealt with in a better way? If YES, please state how.
10. Should any additional information be provided? If YES, please state information required.
11. Was a nurse always available to answer your questions? If NO, please state who was.
12. Do you feel reasonably confident about going home? If NO, please give reasons.
13. Please add any further comments below.

> Day sister: *Well, yes, but quite honestly I think just carry on, because the time we do that and they may not return them. I doubt if we'll ever see them again. We're not giving any advice that shouldn't be in there.*

I raised the need for collaborative practice, which was greeted with some derision. There was a sharing of past experiences of the abrasive public criticism received from some consultants, which had humiliated them and undermined their confidence. As the leaflets were individually devised, the co-researchers felt more vulnerable than if presenting them as a group process.

Patient responses to the leaflets were overall very positive, however the following conversation took place:

> Caroline: *Three patients have now said that my one was too much to read; so I may have to alter it.*
> Benita: *There ought to be more drawings. What was that I read about 83% of the population don't know where their stomach is.*
> Day sister: *Well, I can't draw; there's got to be someone artistic around.*
> Loretta: *Benita can draw; do you remember drawing ... ?*
> Anne: *Yes, Benita you could do one huge drawing of the human body with all the major organs on it.*
> Day sister: *Yes, and we'll stick it somewhere in the ward!* [laughter] *Many people don't know their body at all. Men don't know where their prostates are, no concept of their body at all.*

There was considerable discussion regarding information overload especially if patients were self-medicating and being prepared for PCA. There was much verbal and written information to assimilate on admission. It was possible that in the future the leaflet could be sent to the patient together with the notification for admission letter. The leaflets would also be available in the pre-admission clinic.

Perceptions of the usefulness of the leaflets were highlighted at the nurses' evaluation interviews at the end of the study.

> Fiona: *Even though you have always explained the operation, they now have something to read, and they can give it to their family when they visit for them to read.*

> Geraldine: *I think they are very useful, because they reinforce what you say and give that bit extra information.*
> Benita: *We had one lady, though, who didn't want to look at it. She was very nervous ... we still need to produce many more though.*

At her evaluation interview day sister revealed an interesting outcome:

> Day sister: *They* [leaflets] *have been very well received by the patients, and they seem very happy with them. But it seems as a result of this the Health Authority are now developing booklets on patient information, and I got one in the post yesterday to comment on, and I'm looking at this little printed booklet, and I thought, I've read this somewhere before; this is very familiar. Of course, it's my leaflet on mastectomy, almost word for word ... I'm going to write a note back to them saying it is difficult for me to comment on something that I have actually written!*

Moving forward

To enable a comprehensive appreciation of the three innovations (PSM and drug information leaflets, PCA and the operation-specific leaflets) each has been individually described. To further systematically explore the process and outcomes of nurse-led change and development and how these innovations were perceived, a combined analysis of the group meetings, the innovation evaluations together with the co-researchers' evaluation interviews are discussed in the following chapter.

Chapter 6
Process and outcomes of nurse-led change and development

'Action research enhances and enriches beyond all
imaginings the personal lives of thinking practitioners.'
(McNiff 1988)

The personal and professional development that arose from undertaking the change process is described in this chapter. These outcomes
of the first critical action research study, and the co-researchers'
perceptions of the change process, are derived from an analysis of the
data from the ward group meetings, the co-researchers' interviews and
the patients', co-researchers' and multi-professional team's evaluations
of the three innovations.

Analysis

A variety of texts informed the analytical process. Methods for
analysing qualitative data were drawn from Lofland and Lofland
(1984), Miles and Huberman (1984), Field and Morse (1985), Berg
(1989), Patton (1990) and Riley (1990). To enable familiarity with and
to search for 'surprises' in the data (Riley 1990), the group meetings
were analysed in two ways. First, by coding, category identification and
clustering of categories and, secondly, in combination with the data
from the patient, nurse and multi-professional team evaluations (of the
innovations) and the co-researchers' interviews.

Coding

For the process of coding, I undertook 'open coding' as proposed by Berg (1989), where transcripts are read and all aspects of the content are initially included. I numbered and named sentences or paragraphs from every page of each transcript for later retrieval; these were named as closely as possible to the quotations and behaviours recorded. From the sixteen group meetings, I identified 167 initial codes; these could then be grouped by collapsing the codes to generate categories. Miles and Huberman (1984) refer to this process as data reduction whereby the data is condensed, focused and simplified. Fifty-five categories were identified. Quotations and behaviours that demonstrated each category were placed in individually classified A4-size envelopes. These were then clustered into a final 23 categories.

This process of coding and categorisation spanned many weeks. The data were left and on subsequent occasions re-examined to confirm the appropriateness of classification. Category headings with accompanying relevant examples from the transcripts were cut out, sorted and pasted onto sheets of A3 paper for ease of access. Patton (1990) cautions that, as they do not have statistical tests to tell them when an observation or pattern is significant, qualitative analysts must rely on their own intelligence, experience and judgement. This sometimes leads to the making of the equivalent of Type 1 or Type 2 errors from statistics. The qualitative analyst may decide that something is not significant when in fact it is or, conversely, may attribute significance to something that is meaningless.

The 23 categories which were derived from the group meetings:

Shared reflections   Collaboration
Power conflicts   Knowledge deficit
Initiating action   Humorous coping
Risk-taking   Positive anticipation
Positive reinforcement   Problem-solving
Sharing knowledge   Positive outcomes
Doctors' perceptions   Legal/ethical perspectives
Patients' perspectives   Personal growth
Changing role of the nurse   Reflective analysis
Psychological safety   Shared values
Digression   Time constraints
Feedback avoidance

Managing the data

At this stage I decided that to try to provide a clear explication of the process and outcomes of the study the 23 categories should be analysed in conjunction with the data from the evaluations of the three innovations and the co-researchers' summative evaluations. This reflects Lofland and Lofland's (1984) recommendation of integrating data, interpretation and analysis. This process was facilitated by the theoretical perspectives of critical social science, change theory (as well as motivation theory, experiential learning and reflective practice). The categories identified by Lewin's Force Field Analysis (table 2.1, p. 22) provide an organising framework for the management of the data (table 6.1) and for the descriptive analysis of the process and outcomes of the study (pages 134–161). The headings motivating and modifying factors enabled identification of the process.

Table 6.1: Motivating and modifying factors of the nurse-led change and development process in the practice setting.

Field Analysis	Motivating Factors	Modifying Factors
Technical	Co-researchers' purposeful action Ward manager's collaborative leadership Patient participation	Patients' evaluation, Halo effects
Economic	Assured funding	Time constraints Cost analysis
Political	Doctors' positive perceptions	Power imbalance Power conflicts
Socio-cultural	Humorous coping Action researcher promoting: psychological safety confidence positive anticipation	Digression
Organisational	Managerial validation Empowerment	Managerial goals
Policy	RLT model application	Legal/ethical perspectives
Structural	Bottom-up innovation Collaborative meetings Continuity of meetings	Collaborative practice
Group	Open communication Problem-solving Consensus	Risk-taking

(contd)

Table 6.1: (contd).

Field Analysis	Motivating Factors	Modifying Factors
Interpersonal	Shared values Goal attainment	Feedback avoidance
Individual/personal	Reflective action Process evaluations Personal enhancement	Expectations Self-appraisal Knowledge deficit

The change process evolved from practitioners reflecting on the need to promote psychological independence in their patients (as identified in their nursing model for practice) and planning, implementing and evaluating the resultant innovations.

Co-researchers' evaluation of the study

Semi-structured interviews were undertaken with all the co-researchers fifteen months after the study's inception. Each interview, of 30-45 minutes, was audiotaped. The interviews were undertaken in the patients' sitting room adjacent to the ward; I tried to ensure the utmost privacy. A maximum of two interviews was the most I could undertake in any one day as I became quite emotionally drained by the co-researchers' revelations of their personal and professional development and perceptions of the process and outcomes of the study. The interviews took place over a two-month period.

The semi-structured interview schedule addressed the three innovations: the group meetings, applicability to the RLT model and four items adopted from Fretwell's (1985) evaluation tool related to personal growth and development as a result of the change process (see table 6.2).

Morton-Cooper (2000, 85) believes that the most important criterion for judging an action research study is whether it has cultural validity, that is whether it provides a trustworthy and believable narrative to the practitioner. Bourdieu (1977) cautions that the impulse of interviewees is to recount to the researcher what they think the researcher thinks ought to be occurring, rather than what they think is actually occurring. This is less likely to occur in an action research study as the researcher has been personally involved and has some insight into the effects of the study. I was aware, however, during the first three interviews that when the co-researchers had answered a question I often then gave my opinion. This potential 'leading' could

Table 6.2: Co-researchers' evaluation tool.

PERSONAL INTERVIEW PROFORMA

1. How did the action research study compare with your initial expectations?
2. Of the three innovations, which one has given you the most satisfaction and which the least? Why is that?
3. Has the study made a difference to the way you view your nursing practice? In what ways?
4. How useful were the group sessions? What did you see as being the main focus of the sessions?
5. How did you make the links with the RLT model?
6. Do you feel that this model is useful for surgical nurses? What do you see as the advantages/disadvantages of the RLT model?
7. To what extent did you use your reflective journal?
8. In what ways has being involved in the project helped you?
9. In what ways has being involved in the project hindered you?
10. Are you satisfied/dissatisfied with the way in which you have been involved in the study? Please explain why.
11. What further measures could be taken to facilitate change and bring about a successful outcome to the study?

have influenced later responses during the interview process. It was during transcribing of these interviews that I recognised this unintentioned behaviour. As a result I tried to refrain from comment until the end of each interview. Some of the co-researchers appeared to have greater insight and self-awareness, and each provided, I believe, a realistic evaluation. Much of what they said coincided, and I doubted that they had put a rosier tint on their perceptions of the study.

> Day sister: *It was a lot harder than I thought and took up quite a lot of time as well. I didn't really know what to expect.*
> Hannah: *I thought we would meet a great deal more resentment. I was surprised at how well it did work. I was expecting a lot more hassle.*
> Fiona: *I wasn't sure what to expect. I didn't feel apprehensive. Didn't mind trying anything.*
> Benita: *I was a bit worried because the research bit sounded complicated and very involved. It didn't seem too bad though.*
> Lorraine: *I thought at the beginning, I'm really going to*

enjoy this. It was dynamic and interesting, but I felt we took on too much.
Esther: *It was actually quite enjoyable.*

Descriptive analysis of the process and outcomes of the study

The approach to studying the process and determining outcomes of the study reflects the argument provided by Patton (1990). He states that qualitative inquiry is highly appropriate in studying the process because depicting the process requires detailed description. The experience of process typically varies for different people; process is fluid and dynamic, and participants' perceptions are a key consideration. Such data permits judgements to be made about the extent to which the change process is operating, which enables others not directly involved in the study to understand the process. By describing and understanding the dynamics of the process, it is possible to isolate critical elements that have contributed to the successes and failures of the study.

Measurable goals are often specified to determine outcomes. However, Patton (1990) advocates that, as individuals may identify varying process outcomes, the unique meaning of that outcome for each person should be documented. Within the action research cycle there may be difficulty in specifying outcomes as, by its nature, new problems arise which then require further problem-solving, action planning, implementation and evaluation. The problem then, according to Webb (1993), is to determine the point in time when a process ceases to be a process activity and becomes an outcome. Consequently the factors indicative of the innovative change process have been identified (table 6.1 and below) and a combined descriptive account of these factors and the perceived outcomes undertaken. The perceived outcomes for the patients, the co-researchers, the NUM, the action researcher and the organisation are also addressed.

Interpersonal - Shared values

It would be difficult to determine a hierarchy of motivating factors for this study. Nevertheless our shared values and beliefs should be viewed as highly significant. Nolan and Grant (1993) assert that establishing the basic values that underpin the care in a given area should be the first stage of an action research study. The responses to the RLT self-rating scale and the process of agreement established in the feedback meeting (chapter 4) had, in some part, addressed this stage. My past relationship with most of the co-researchers had reinforced our shared perspectives.

Johnson (1990) notes that communication of new ideas is more effective and more comfortable among those who share common attributes such as values, beliefs, education and professional interests. According to Rogers (1983) such homophily can act as an invisible barrier to the flow of innovations within a system, causing new ideas to flow horizontally among like-minded individuals (rather than vertically across career paths within a profession). Our sharing of explicit (and implicit?) personal values therefore enhanced the development of the change process.

No formal values-clarification exercise was initiated in this study. It may have caused some difficulty, embarrassment and/or resentment, especially amongst the more reserved of the co-researchers. I felt a less structured approach would enhance collaborative agreement and practice. Rogers (1989) notes that for many nurses having an opportunity to discuss the meaning of nursing and to talk about their beliefs, values and assumptions is a new experience.

> Jane: *Well, what was important to me was finding out what other people's feelings were. Sitting and talking all together rather than just a one to one.*
> Hannah: *Actually, being able to sit down and talk about nursing. You don't have time on the ward to find out how others seriously feel about things.*

To the NUM the difficulty and dilemma of balancing bureaucratic demands of cost-costing and budgeting with professional priorities was in evidence:

> *I think if I costed it out* [PCA] *I probably wouldn't be allowed to continue with it, but people* [non-nurse managers] *do tend to look at the sums and don't look at the other end, at the patient, and that's why I have held off a little bit.*

Views of patients, both positive and negative, were shared. These sometimes conflicted with the right to respect the patient's wishes and prompt the question: do patients always know what is best for them?

> Fiona: *Patients are not always honest, are they? They're certainly not liked by everyone. You should have the right not to like everyone but to still respect them.*

> Caroline: *Patients don't always know what's best for them. It's important to help patients do as much as they can for themselves to enable them to go home as soon as possible especially with the old dears. You should encourage them even when they say they don't want to. We persuaded Mrs M. to walk down the ward. She was so chuffed. It was wonderful after what she had been through.*
> Night sister: *We need to change the wording there* [on the protocol] *because you might be cutting a lot of people out. I mean the traveller, for example.*
> Caroline: *The 92-year-old lady who had the mastectomy liked the leaflet.*
> Denise: *She was wonderful. She looked great, and she just told us what to do.* [laughs]
> Geraldine: *It just goes to show that age doesn't come into it.*
> Esther: *Yes; they're all individuals.*

However, ethical dilemmas occurred, which challenged the belief in a patient's right to choose. Malin and Teasdale (1991) note that unresolved tensions exist between the choice of empowering interventions and the employment of more protective, caring approaches. I referred to the sister of a nursing development unit who had implemented PSM.

> Loretta: *Now she believes that it's up to the patient whether they wish to lock it* [their bedside drug cabinet] *or not, would we consider doing this?*

D'Crutz and Bottoff (1984) believe that it is through a supportive emotional atmosphere of interpersonal involvement that a holistic approach in nursing can be achieved. These shared perspectives may be viewed as examples of this approach and what Salvage (1990) has termed the 'new nursing', attempting to replace the traditional relationship of dominant expert and passive client with that of a more egalitarian form of interaction, which promotes active patient participation.

Technical - Leadership style

The ward manager's collaborative leadership style was vital for the development of change and the implementation of the action research cycle. She shared her knowledge and her lack of it, valued the nurses as individuals and encouraged group decision-making. Dunham and Fisher (1990) find that empowerment requires recognising staff potential and unleashing that potential to accompany the vision.

> Day sister: *Well, now we all need to decide who we're going to push it out to first* [the PSM protocol] *... Is there any reason why P., S., and J.* [health care assistants] *can't reinforce things? Because they've often got more time than we have, and they'll feel part of it as well ... I think perhaps sometimes I find it hard to devolve things to others, but I do try.*
> NUM: (evaluation interview): *I put it down to M.* [day sister] *. She involves everybody, and if you do that, you get that commitment and everybody has got something to offer. And you can see them constantly pushing one another. They constantly want things, which is good. It is down to the leadership that they get and the fact that they are all involved.*

For example, when the co-researchers were slow to ask patients to evaluate their devised operation-specific information leaflets:

> Day sister: *I mean, it's up to us - we've got to do it; if we don't, it's a wasted exercise.*

Organisational - Managerial perspective

Support from the NUM was integral to the study and was demonstrated by validating the co-researchers' initiatives and financial expenditure and by becoming personally involved in the implementation process. She had been in post for approximately four months when phase 1 commenced and initially felt ambivalence towards the study. She had acknowledged her staff's proposals, however, rather than advocate her own agenda:

> *I know that initially it was quite difficult for me. I wanted to come up with some of my ideas, but then I took a step back and thought you know what it is about, it has got to be from them and whatever will come will be of benefit. I can remember feeling a little bit aggrieved; I wished I could do what I want to.*

The supportive role that she adopted empowered the nurses to effect change. It provided them with emancipatory support - the freedom to identify and to implement the changes in practice. The process had enabled her to value the practitioners' perspectives and priorities of care:

> *I think I feel so far removed now in some ways that you forget that one of the things you did was take control of patients. And looking back now has made me remember what it was like when I was doing it* [bedside nursing] *every day. And I suppose that, yes, it is top priority, but at my level it would not have been. An eye opener for me.*

The need for nurse managers to empower their staff by enabling them to 'release their creativity, talent and vision in order to enhance nursing and healthcare' is proposed by Watson-Druee (1994). She suggests that nurse managers (who are also leaders) will feel empowered when other nurses are empowered. One important principle in this transformational leadership process is for managers to give visibility to others and provide recognition for their efforts:

> NUM:*This ward is now used as a resource. The rest of the hospital are very interested in what has been happening on PSM now it is up and running and with PCA too. When someone phones me to say they have a patient returned from theatre with PCA, who wasn't prepared, and what should they do, I tell them to contact a member of Ward A. I've told them how good, very good they are at educating both patients and staff.*

Group - Empowerment

The concept of empowerment, of power sharing and freedom of choice, for both patients and co-researchers was a powerful motivator for change. The co-researchers' aim was to promote optimum psychological independence for their patients by enabling 'appropriate' patients to have some control over their situation by electing to participate in their care.

> Jane: *I want to inform them more about what is going on. It's amazing that people don't know what their tablets are for or why they are having an operation.*

Empowering patients, however, raises legal and ethical issues. The rights of patients to decline PSM, PCA and receive written operation details are acknowledged. However, for some, patient choice has to be tempered by selection criteria to ensure their safety and comfort: the nurse's duty of care.

> Lorraine: *It was very difficult for me trying to explain to a patient who up until admission was taking their own tablets that now I didn't think they could manage.*

The positive feedback from the patients increased the co-researchers' motivation for change in spite of the 'halo effect/angels' perspective colouring some patients' judgements.

> Day sister: *It has definitely made a lot of them* [patients] *more questioning about what the tablets are for and why they are taking them and should they take this one with that one; so I think that has been good for the patients.*
> Fiona: *Most of the patients seem really pleased with it* [self-medication]. *They were quite chuffed that they could do it themselves.*
> Jane: *I think patients are really pleased with PCA and self-medication; they are more in control. I also gave them the evaluation questionnaire thing for my leaflet. They wrote they were pleased with it and glad to have something to refer to when going home.*

In their study on nurse-patient interactive styles Krouse and Roberts (1989) conclude that interaction should be evaluated on variables such as feelings of control, power and satisfaction. Feelings of power and control over one's destiny may also be found to influence factors such as compliance with treatment, following of other health practices and a general sense of satisfaction with health professionals (Chang et al. 1994).

Empowering of staff is a current yet controversial issue. Mackenzie's (1993) study reveals that a quarter of the sisters/charge nurses (n = 93) did not feel free to make autonomous decisions on clinical and professional matters, and East and Robinson (1993) find that many ward sisters who wanted to make changes seemed blocked at every turn and that they felt like victims of organisational forces over which they had no control. Hayward et al. (1991) identify staff nurses' feelings of disempowerment, and Grant et al. (1994) see these as a reflection of the management style and also as a result of the welter of changes affecting the nursing profession and the NHS. These perceptions were not in evidence regarding this change process:

> Hannah: *We would all have an idea and then knock it out together.*
> Benita: *We ironed out the problems of what was going wrong then we were able to put things right.*
> Fiona: *Basically, I've enjoyed being involved in something that we actually got off the ground, and it actually seems to benefit the patients and is nice for us as well that they have mastered it. We need to keep it going now that we have actually got it going.*
> Caroline: *I feel quite satisfied. Being part-time, I didn't feel I got so actively involved, but it worked out well because we all wanted to do it and we were given the opportunity to do it.*

Group - Dynamics

At many group meetings the costs and benefits of the innovations were debated. This risk analysis was facilitated by open communication, group problem-solving and consensus. Open communication enabled us to share our knowledge and also to highlight our strengths and deficits, undertake judicious planning and receive feedback as constructive criticism. I tried to pre-plan the meetings, which always consisted of an update and feedback exchange of information, setting priorities, reviewing the time-scale, action plans and deployment of tasks. There had to be flexibility in the structure and continuity of the meetings (which lasted approximately one hour) to enable group reflection and group strategies such as action planning and devising evaluation tools.

> Lorraine: *The group sessions were very, very useful. Things that you think are silly then you find that other people have the same problems. I think we gave each other a lot of confidence. We all got together and found ways round the problems, whereas one person probably wouldn't have been able to do it ... everyone had their say.*

Group planning and problem-solving were key features. The group became more cohesive as the study progressed.

> Day sister: *I felt once they got used to the group idea it brought out people who might normally have said nothing. I thought some quite good ideas came out of it. They all agreed to do things, and they actually did it.*
> Fiona: *They were good especially for a moan. We looked into how to solve problems ... everybody's input was considered.*

The frequent meetings appeared to provide an appropriate environment for consistent dynamic group interaction. There is a dearth of literature, however, which addresses the facilitation process of action research meetings. Indeed nurse action researchers appear to focus on the antecedents of their projects. Webb (1989) and Meyer (1993b) describe in depth the problematic process of creating the appropriate group dynamics for change.

> Until staff are able to work together comfortably there will be no point in trying to introduce [appropriate group dynamics for change]. Indeed a collaborative and supportive atmosphere is the essential foundation for motivation and commitment to change. (Webb 1989, 131)
> Throughout the study the findings from interviews and field notes revealed a team reluctant to change, lacking cohesion and exhibiting all the signs of dynamic conservatism. (Meyer 1993b)

As a co-researcher I contributed to group discussion and problem-solving but often only after all the other nurses' input. I believe that action planning should be initiated whenever possible by the practitioners. My input was often to generate responses, for example:

> *How are we going to evaluate self-medication? ... So here's my inevitable question, what are you going to do about it? ... I'll read out this leaflet* [drug information] *and please all comment.*

The co-researchers decided to continue with the group meetings for ongoing problem-solving and support after I withdrew from the study.

Socio-cultural - Coping

Two coping strategies which were often in evidence at the meetings were humorous coping and digression.

> Day sister (evaluation interview): *We tend to digress a lot, which is normal for us lot on here.* [laughs]

Humour and laughter have been identified as aiding in stress reduction by decreasing task anxiety and improving cognitive retention and task performance (Smith et al. 1971), and allowing objective self-analysis without losing face (Williams 1986 in Astedt-Kurki and Liukkonen 1994). According to Dossey and Keegan (1988) and Parrott (1994), as nursing can be extremely challenging, rewarding and stressful, humour is seen as a necessary tool for one's ability to maintain some semblance of sanity in often sobering or bizarre settings.

> Loretta: *Well, you do have a lot of knowledge; I've said this before, but you don't always realise it.*
> Denise: *Yes, it's amazing because you normally can answer patients' queries.*
> Hannah: *What you mean like what's a bedpan?*

Much of the digression was related to the ward rather than social events and often addressed the co-researchers' changing roles.

> Denise: *But we just seem to be taking things off the doctors' shoulders at the moment ... it's detracting from what we're doing as nurses as they're cutting their hours down.*
> Fiona: *We're now doing phlebotomy, ECGs, IVs, where does nursing come into it?*
> [much heated discussion]:
> Day sister: *I haven't been to break today, nor yesterday nor the day before ... People are tearing their hair out trying to do 24 hours work into eight hours; we must look at 24-hour care. Now we'll get back to you, Loretta.*
> Caroline: *We'll need stress workshops soon.*
> Loretta: *Well, I could do that.*
> Denise: *Yes, that would be great, and you could come in here without that tape recorder on!*

It was on these occasions that I felt the most uncomfortable. I could try to empathise but felt these changes were adding untimely additional stresses to the co-researchers. It was difficult to gauge the extent to which the innovations could be jeopardised by these critical demands. Non-malicious laughter and flippant remarks were directed at patients, members of the multi-professional team and at one another. We all benefited from this emotional release, or catharsis, which was a feature of many meetings. This was also no doubt due to the pressure of implementing three initiatives in quick succession together with working in an acute care setting. The caution by Webb was extremely pertinent at this time:

> Only one change should be introduced at a time, and evaluated and modified as necessary. Only when this was established practice should another change be tried. (1989, 124)

There is no right time to implement change in a dynamic clinical environment, but there are conditions which can advance the process, hence the identification of the motivating factors in table 6.1. Nevertheless, it may be that initiating an action research study should be considered in the midst of political and organisational change. It provides an open format for group discussion and support and enables the powerless group to initiate their own agenda for change. Consequently, this strategy could empower nurses to become more proactive, to define their current and future roles, rather than succumb to political and professional forces.

Individual - Reflective action

Reflection is an implicit part of the action research cycle (pages 24–26). Prerequisites to reflection include open-mindedness and motivation (Boud et al. 1985, Goodman 1989). Atkins and Murphy (1993) believe that reflection must involve the self and must lead to a changed perspective; this they say is one crucial aspect which distinguishes reflection from analysis. Two of the innovations, PSM and PCA, emerged from the group reflecting on everyday practice situations and the concept of independence/dependence (RLT model). Individual motivation appeared in part to be linked to reflecting on individual creative application of each innovation, which was articulated at the group meetings.

The co-researchers agreed to commence writing personal reflections. However, in reality this was rarely undertaken. They adapted the focused structured reflection tool that I had provided to facilitate the process for their own needs (page 98). However, I was aware that very little reflective writing was being undertaken and reasoned that I had provided inadequate preparation. The ego-protective function, as described by Argyris and Schon (1974), and the implicitness of much of nursing practice may also have contributed to this situation. On occasions I alluded to this strategy:

> *Well, if you haven't written anything in your reflective journal recently, maybe now might be the time with PCA about to happen.*

In fact very little was actually written in any of the journals during phase two. The reasons given were very similar. Even though I stated from the outset that the journals were private and no one was to see them, committing their reflections to paper was either viewed as painful and threatening or too difficult, and in the main unnecessary, for these clinical practitioners, because there was good social support within the group (see table 6.3).

Table 6.3: Co-researchers' perceptions of reflective journals.

Informant	To what extent did you use your reflective journal?
Day sister	Very little, I'm afraid. I couldn't quite see the relevance. As nurses, we mentally reflect without writing it down. We have not been brought up with reflective diaries, whereas the students coming through now have to write it all down.
Lorraine	Not really, verbally it is not a problem but to put it in writing ... If it was a negative incident, would I really want to read about it at a later date? All the stress and pain I might feel would come rushing back, too depressing.
Jane	I didn't have one from the start [laughs]. You forgot to give me one!
Hannah	I hid a photograph in it. I wrote a bit about PCA, but I don't really like writing things down, and I certainly can't look at it again. I find it a threat because someone could read it, and I don't think any of us really want anyone else to know what we are thinking. It is too much of me ... I am as open as I will ever be, and that's more than an awful lot of people I know.
Fiona	I put a few things in it, feelings that bothered me. I suppose it's useful if you document an incident and then you have to go to court or something. Well, you can look back to see what

	you thought about it, but you'd probably feel different about it a couple of months later.
Benita	I did think about it, but I didn't actually write anything down … because no one else was doing it. I think that if people had done it I might feel guilty.
Caroline	Once, not touched it apart from that once. It nearly got me into trouble. My husband said: 'What's in this book?' I told him to put it back in the drawer. I find it difficult to write things down. I think I reflect anyway. I don't need to put it in black and white.
Denise	I didn't write in it at all. I really wanted to, but when it actually came to sitting there putting pen to paper … it's like listening to yourself on tape: it could be embarrassing for you.
Esther	I didn't use it at all. I think we reflect anyway on the ward. I suppose that sometimes I don't even think about what I have done … just do them automatically, don't think about them. I would rather go to the social club and have a drink with the girls and reflect in that way.
Geraldine	I didn't do it. Writing it down for me is not the easiest thing to do anyway … but working with the girls here we go out for a drink, good or rough times we always talk about it. If I was to write something down, I'd be conscious that someone might read it … I don't see the point really.

The negative perceptions of self-reflective writing did not, however, appear to detract from the group reflective behaviours, which the co-researchers highly favoured, and which met their needs for the reflective process of the action research cycle. Each co-researcher was very satisfied with the outcome of the study, fulfilling the characteristics of experiential learning (Kolb 1984) - a concrete experience, observation and reflection, abstract conceptualisation and putting into practice. Certainly reflection on action (Schon 1991) was evident at the meetings. This was initially seen by reflecting on the concept of psychological independence, which led to the identification of PSM and PCA from everyday nursing situations; reflecting on personal feedback from patients, peers, and members of the multi-professional team and verbalised self-reflections on action. Individual and group analysis and personal creativity led to the application of the outcomes of reflection in practice, i.e. reflective action.

The keeping of a reflective journal, supported by a facilitator, may enable a practitioner to critically analyse and evaluate their experiences and enhance their self-awareness. Yet this strategy may be considered inappropriate where nurses have social support and are able to share their critical perspectives of nursing and offload onto their peers.

The skills of reflection (whether written or oral) incorporate the process of perspective transformation (Mezirow 1981) whereby current perspectives are critically analysed and new perspectives give rise to fundamental structural changes in the way individuals see themselves and their relationships with others, leading to a reinterpretation of their personal, social or occupational worlds. Perspective transformation is comparable with empowerment theory:

> In becoming empowered, individuals are not merely acquiring new practical skills; they are reconstructing and reorientating deeply ingrained personal systems of social relations. Moreover they confront these tasks in an environment which historically has enforced their 'political' repression and which continues its active and implicit attempts at subversion of constructive change. However, it is not simply the issue of time that is so crucial, but more importantly the question of practice. Empowerment is not a commodity to be acquired, but a transforming process constructed through action. Throughout the proposed development model, reflective experience is the irreducible source of growth.
> (Kieffer 1987 in Johns 1993, 16)

Individual - Personal enhancement

Personal enhancement in nursing can be linked to job satisfaction. According to Cavanagh (1992), there are three main reasons why this is a vital area for study. Nursing is a very stressful occupation, and therefore intrinsic satisfaction can act as a counterbalance by providing moments of reward. Job satisfaction can potentially influence patient care, and job satisfaction impinges on organisational issues (particularly those relating to job turnover and staff morale). Examples related to these three reasons can be extrapolated from the co-researchers' perceptions of the outcomes of the study (see table 6.4).

Table 6.4: Co-researchers' perceptions of personal advantages and disadvantages of the study.

Informant	How has the study helped you?	How has the study hindered you?
Day sister	Made me think more about traditional practices. Able to develop my writing. I could relate what I was learning (undertaking Diploma in Nursing); so that was brilliant.	I suppose only timewise really. I worried about leaving the ward a bit short when we had the meetings and having to use my own time at home.
Lorraine	Broadened my knowledge and motivated me to do other things. I now want to do a counselling course. It has certainly made me try to spend even more time explaining things to patients.	It hasn't. I quite enjoyed it all. All the extra reading too, which was very helpful.
Jane	It has made me want to carry on studying ... It was good to have the chance to learn all the new things that were going on and to do something different.	I can't think of anything.
Hannah	Better understanding and definitely helped me to get on with my work. I'm even more aware of treating people as individuals ... To look at nursing moving forward rather than: 'Oh good, I've got a child; let's relax!'	So much paperwork. Not so much all the typing I did but can take a long time going through all the paperwork with the patients.
Fiona	I assess patients better now and have learnt to trust them more. I try to give them more of my time rather than rushing around all the time. It gave me something to work for rather than just poodling along day after day.	Probably just the time factor.

(contd)

Table 6.4: (contd).

Informant	How has the study helped you?	How has the study hindered you?
Benita	I've learnt that you do need to use everybody to get something going well. I have offered to do a lecture with Geraldine now. I would never have done that in the past! It's really made me look at pain control. Everybody should be considered a potential candidate for PCA.	Not going home on Thursdays [group meetings day]! I can't think of anything else except I have to try not to forget to give out all the forms.
Caroline	Feel more of a team. It's also a good feeling to be up to date, even one step ahead. I look at patients more as individuals. I feel I have even more of a rapport with patients now.	I felt lost at times because of being part-time. When I came back to work after three days it was that bit harder to remember all that was going on.
Denise	It has made the work interesting. It has made me feel proud to work on here. It helps your confidence too. It makes you realise how good it is to bring new things in and how difficult it is as well. It highlighted that so many people do not know anything about their tablets, quite amazing.	No, not at all. The extra work we needed to do anyway. There is no point in just coming in and doing the minimum and going home; it's nice to stretch yourself and do a bit more anyway. You might think: 'I have got to write about that drug', but at least when you have done it you feel good about it and feel positive.
Esther	It has given me more confidence in myself. I am now looking at pain control in terminally ill patients ... You think about drugs and side effects more, before you just dished them out ... Now I physically sit and go through their drugs with them, whereas normally I probably wouldn't have thought about it, to be honest.	I don't think it has really.

Table 6.4: (contd).

Informant	How has the study helped you?	How has the study hindered you?
Geraldine	Being aware that you can change things. I felt good to be part of such a team, we worked well ... We all had our equal share of things to do, I liked the way we were all equally involved. Learnt a lot about drugs. It's been great.	It has been hard work at times, but you've just got to put these things in front of you.

The NUM summarised her thoughts about the changes in the co-researchers' personal and professional development:

> NUM: *I can see when I come on the ward - the change. It is automatic now. Dealing with PSM and teaching all about it, and explaining it all, and do they want the PCA after their operation, and they sit there and they go through the whole procedure with them. To see them sitting and teaching the patients, the bond is starting very early on. It seems to break down barriers a lot quicker with the patients.*

These positive outcomes of the study may be categorised as:

Personal enhancement:

- increased knowledge-base
- improved written and verbal communication skills
- increased teaching skills
- sense of achievement
- increased confidence
- motivated to undertake further study

Patient-centred enhancement:

- linked theory to practice
- greater insight into nursing practice

Group enhancement:

- greater team cohesion

Empowerment:

- questioned the status quo
- provided achievable goals
- felt able to make changes

The Audit Commission (1991) states that managers will have to engage in a fundamental rethink of ways in which job satisfaction can be increased through better management and changing patterns of care. The desirable changes in the co-researchers were viewed as highly significant by the NUM.

> NUM: *I think it has been difficult, more difficult than I would initially have thought, but I wouldn't think their enthusiasm has dipped; it has been fairly constant and kept coming and that is important. There have been problems, especially with PCA; yet none of them has altered or felt we will go back. They still want to keep going until we get it right. The night staff too all wanted to take it on. They are not going to let it go back; they want it to continue, and they are each trying to fine tune it, which I think is good.*

Economic - Time constraints

Time constraints have cost implications but are inevitable when undertaking research in a dynamic clinical setting. Time constraints were linked to four main areas:

- trying to efficiently manage the one-hour group meetings
- the problems that delayed implementation of PSM and PCA
- the ability of the co-researchers to attend the meetings and to incorporate new working practices into their span of duty
- the deadline for completion of the study

Although there was some loose structure to the group meetings, time had to be made available for all the co-researchers to feed back their observations and to enable group reflection and problem-solving. The meeting rarely started on time. By around 1415 hours most staff would be present, but then I felt we needed to have a few minutes to socialise and unwind. The co-researchers often attended in their off-duty time, this was always the case for the night nurses (although evening meetings had been suggested too, but the night staff seemed quite happy with the arrangement). There were often interruptions as the seminar room where the meetings took place was adjacent to the ward and on occasions a nurse would have to (understandably) leave the meeting to attend to a patient or speak to a relative or doctor. Nurses who were unable to leave patients for the start of the meeting often managed to pop in at some stage. I began to wonder if chaos theory might have provided a more appropriate theoretical framework!

> Caroline: (evaluation interview) *Finding the time to attend was difficult; you felt sometimes you really should have stayed in the ward because of the pressure of work ... but to do it at all you had to make the effort to attend. It certainly improved our team work in the ward.*

Trying to predict the impact of the innovations on the working day was a common feature of the meetings.

> Anne: *How much more time do you think it* [self-medication] *will take when you admit someone?*

The problems that delayed PSM and PCA are discussed on pages 109, 110, 119 and 120. Although I had emphasised the importance of good planning, after three months, some of the co-researchers were wanting some action:

> Geraldine: *It seems so slow.*
> Loretta: *Well, it's not so slow is it? We only really started it all off in February. Where are we now? May, a lot's been done, especially when you think how busy the ward is.*

My frustration was also evident, owing to delaying the implementation of the innovations. One of the co-researchers (Caroline) had adopted a more realistic assessment of the situation.

> Loretta to Caroline: *You did say this wasn't going to start until September didn't you? So we can't start; obviously we can't start until everything's ready; so we'll have to delay a little, not for long hopefully, else I couldn't bear it.*

Political - Power issues

At the start of phase 2 many issues that the co-researchers reflected on were often associated with doctor-nurse communications rather than directly related to a patient. These were usually stressful events where the co-researchers described feelings of powerlessness:

> Night sister: *I don't normally get angry at work, but, when you have been nursing for some time and feel relatively confident and the junior doctor just ignores your advice, something like this just makes you feel totally out of control of the situation.*

I felt that to enable the study to develop it was important for the co-researchers to be able to get these stressful events off their chest. At the group meetings I asked them to reflect on their actions if they again encountered a similar situation. Their colleagues provided psychological support and offered advice.

Feelings of powerlessness related to the three innovations were frequently displayed at the group meetings (see pages 107, 120 and 127); yet they were often unfounded. These feelings reflected a low sense of self-worth and the fear of ridicule and rejection of their creativity from a powerfully influential group. Speedy (1989) claims that nurses think of themselves as second-class citizens and lack self-esteem. Rogers (1989) asserts that many nurses are not consciously aware of, nor do they value, their nursing knowledge and their capacity to affect the health of people. Nurses tend to value medical knowledge more highly. (This could be one of the reasons why many nurses may still prefer a medical model as their conceptual model for practice, see chapter 3).

A key problem from the analysis of the data, although never articulated, was the co-researchers' fear of criticism of their writing ability. This was particularly related to their reluctance to send the consultants the protocol and the operation-specific leaflets. (They had also not written in the reflective journals.) The co-researchers' coping strategy resulted in feedback avoidance, a form of denial. Patronis Jones (1994) notes that more multidisciplinary approaches to care are being implemented and investigated without a total understanding of what occurs between two disciplines, nursing and medicine. Verbal communications were far less of a problem.

> Day sister: *Well, C.* [NUM] *was saying today to ask Mr S.* [surgeon] *as a lot of his patients would be suitable*

> *candidates* [for PCA]. *I'll go and see him. I'm sure he won't have any objections.*

It was hoped that by participating in critical action research the co-researchers would feel more confident in their own abilities which would then enable them to initiate and implement further innovation by working in a more collaborative way with medical staff. Fry et al. (1994) believe that nurses are no longer submissive powerless people; nursing is learning to value itself as its own best resource.

Structural - Collaborative practice

> Co-operation between nurse managers, clinical nurses, researchers and educators is not optional but a necessity in order to achieve optimum healthcare for patients. (Lorentzon 1993, 43)

There was open communication and co-operation amongst and between the co-researchers, the NUM and myself. Collaborative practice, initially in the form of co-operation, was also undertaken with pharmacists, doctors and the legal department. According to Weiss (1985), nurses do not find collaboration with physicians and patients an effective or possible behavioural strategy. Yet, by implementing and evaluating the three innovations with patients, the co-researchers had demonstrated collaborative practice. There were, however, problems with anaesthetists in the implementation of PCA. I can only surmise as to the reasons for this resistance to change. Yet Rubright (1984) cautions that physicians have differing priorities, opposing constituencies and individual personality distinctions. He advises:

> Building the confidence and co-operation of physicians so that they will engage in team activities with others in the hospital will require that the team objectives are ones with which they agree, the rules of the game are acceptable, and there is a valuable and publicised end result. (Rubright 1984)

Feelings of powerlessness were evident:

> Jane: *We explain it* [PCA] *to them* [patients]*; yet they don't always come back with it. It's not in our hands*

> *really I suppose. All we can do is explain and hope that*
> *they* [anaesthetists] *will do it.*

The day sister reinforced the PCA administration process by meeting with one of the anaesthetists, and I wrote to them all explaining the problem and the effects on both patients and staff. I asked them to contact me to discuss the issue further, but none responded. Lenkman and Gribbins (1994) caution that multi-professional teamwork cannot be achieved overnight and will require a substantial commitment to education, empowerment, and autonomy in decision-making at all levels throughout the organisation from the board down to the most recently hired employee. Collaborative practice with other members of the multi-professional team was evident.

> Night sister (clarifying roles, to the pharmacist): *I need to*
> *be sure of the role of the ward pharmacist in all this.*
> *How far does your accountability extend?*
> Loretta: *Well, I mean pharmacy should be as co-opera-*
> *tive as possible as the ward pharmacist, S., has been*
> *involved right from the start.*

Yet the district pharmacist had added to the PSM protocol without informing the ward pharmacist or the co-researchers:

> Hannah: *Now, here's a bit not in the original. That*
> *pharmacy may not be able to support individual supplies*
> *of all drugs to patients who are self-medicating. That bit*
> *has been slipped in.*
> Benita: *That sounds like a cop out.*
> Jane: *Well, it won't work then will it if they only supply*
> *half the medications?*

Collaborative practice did not always occur with their peers:

> Day sister: *Well, we send our patients down with their*
> *nursing care plans, they're* [Recovery nurses] *supposed*
> *to write in them, but half the time they never get done.*
> Hannah: *I've asked down there a couple of times why*
> *they don't give pain control, but I just get a mouthful!*

Collaborative information received by the co-researchers was critically analysed. Reviewers suggested helpful additions to the patient information part of the protocol (for PSM), but night sister commented on the suggestion from the legal department:

> Night sister: *I don't want to put anyone down but how helpful is the word concept for patients?*

Sociocultural - Action researcher

> The atmosphere in an effective group tends to be relaxed and informal, with each member feeling accepted and valued. (Dashiff in Lancaster and Lancaster 1982, 60)

My participation in the process and outcome of change was that of creating and building a trusting relationship within the group, facilitating individual support and collaboration, and contributing to discussion and the sharing of knowledge, risk analysis, action planning and evaluation. I tried to create a psychologically safe environment to enable open communication for, as Drummond (1977 in Meleis and Burton 1981, 37) points out, the most significant element in the change process and implementation of an innovation 'is not the plan of action, nor the objectives, nor the evaluation schema, but rather those plans dealing with human interactions during the stress periods associated with the change'.

> Loretta: *This article talks about sharing fears and worries with peers. This is the nature of support, we all need it.*
> Geraldine: *Everyone felt involved. We went through our leaflets, and no one was made to feel stupid.*

I also found that one of my key roles was that of motivator. I tried to achieve this by promoting confidence and positive anticipation. I was known to most of the co-researchers because I had been the (clinical link) lecturer to the ward. I had, however, only been involved in facilitating student-nurse practice; so it was a challenge, an enriching learning experience, but above all a privilege to facilitate clinical practitioners in innovative change.

Motivation - Promoting confidence

> Your practical expertise, your extensive knowledge, you are moving along this line ... Whatever is generated here will be valuable, very valuable and should be shared to enhance our knowledge of nursing ... Everyone will

have looked and commented on the protocol. I feel it's a formality to go to the Drug and Therapeutics Committee. I mean that's how I see it, and I don't know if they want to be heavy-handed, but whatever they say I personally don't think they would make too many changes. They couldn't come back at this stage and say you've got to make major changes because it's obvious that you've thought it through in great detail ... Has everyone seen the glowing letter from Mr Y.? [consultant surgeon praising PSM, see page 108]. *So I want to work this through* [patients signing drug charts] *for your benefit as well as the patients' ... What we need to do is look at how confident you feel about patient teaching. What are the sorts of things you teach already? ... So that's very positive; we are well on the way ... I'll find it very interesting to hear how you give the information to patients and what sort of reception you get.*[laughter]

Day sister: *Do you think that's all right as a general protocol?*

Loretta: *Yes, I think it's fine. I don't have a problem.*

Day sister: *Oh good.*

Day sister: *It's going to take a long time, and I can see they'll be lots of hiccoughs.*

Loretta: *That's often the way with innovations. You have to look long term.*

Loretta: *I just know I'll miss the start of it* [PSM] *as I'll be on leave.*

NUM: *That's a shame.*

Loretta: *No, not really; you don't need me; I've got great faith in you all.*[laughter]

Motivation - Promoting positive anticipation

The group will decide what action it wants to take. If you feel that there is an issue that needs addressing, we can all try to solve the problem, and then we can implement the strategy and evaluate it. It's not going to be discussion and that's it ... Fine, well that's exciting, isn't it? Will there be many people here to make the choice? [locking medicine cabinets] *... Can we start the meeting folks? Good, I want us to make some decisions today ...*

> *It'll be interesting to see how many we get back* [patient leaflet evaluation forms]. *Interesting to look at them ... Let's be positive about this,* [commencing self-medication], *if there are changes, hopefully they'll only be minor ones.* [laughter] *... It would probably take you a day* [to write the protocol], *but you all need to get together to do it. When you distribute it, identify a date for return. If they're not returned by then, that's tough ... It'll be interesting in a couple of weeks' time, won't it, because I anticipate there'll be far more patients self-medicating. C.* [NUM] *was saying that the other wards are keen to get started; so you'll be the experts.*

At one meeting I related the telephone conversation that I had had with the sister of a ward who had implemented PSM. She cautioned that explaining drugs to a patient could be a very time-consuming process. I responded: 'Well, we've developed drug information leaflets. She said: "Oh, that's a good idea; why didn't I think of that!"'

> Night sister: *You need to be happy that they know what they* [drugs] *are all for.*
> Loretta: *I mean, it'll be quite good because you'll all be learning about the drugs and getting more information from patients as well.*

There were times, however, when I was unable to sustain a positive perspective; this was mainly because of time constraints.

> *Well, I've typed up the evaluation forms for when it* [PCA] *takes off. Keep them on the ward, and, if it ever gets off the ground, there's one for patients and one for staff. Hopefully, by the next meeting at least one person will have given out their* [operation-specific] *leaflet, because it would be good to have some feedback ... Maybe I can arrange fortnightly meetings for support from the end of September* [because of PSM's two months' slippage], *but it's going to be difficult for me.*

The NUM valued my support, whereas I appeared ambivalent about my role, because I would have liked to have had more time to work alongside the co-researchers on the ward. My post limited my access to the clinical area.

> NUM: *I was really pleased with the project. Very impressed with it all. Without your support, I don't think it would have got off the ground.*
> Loretta: *I only helped to pull it all together, a facilitator. It is a positive outcome, but you never know with action research which way it is going to go. I think we were all so committed at the end of the day.*

Being on the fringe, however, did have its advantages. From a more detached viewpoint, I had a wider perspective - 'the onlooker sees all'. I was not constrained by the stresses of the ward, and, although I could empathise with them, the co-researchers' problems did not directly affect me. When the co-researchers therefore were frustrated and tired and wondering if PSM and PCA would ever take off, I was able to stand back and identify positive indicators and direct progress. I do, however, agree with Webb's (1993, 133) assertion that sometimes action researchers certainly do not know where they are going: it is only when they have reached a certain point that they will be able to understand what has been happening.

Policy - RLT application

The perceptions of each co-researcher regarding the application of the RLT model is demonstrated in table 6.5. At the time only day sister had undertaken any form of higher education in nursing studies: 'I can certainly make the links, but I don't know how the others will view that as they haven't had the same teaching that I've had recently.'

These responses demonstrate varying levels of knowledge and conceptualisation. I had assumed as the study developed that the co-researchers would have made strong links with the model. Yet there had been no time at the group meetings to explore this aspect. I was hoping, however, that by using the tool for structured reflection adapted for the RLT model, and the reflective journal, that the co-researchers would have produced significant examples of application to practice based on the innovations. The journals were rarely used however. Yet, when exploring how useful the model was for them, the surgical nurses all felt it was of significant benefit as it was 'simple to use ... an appropriate assessment and evaluation tool'. However, three co-researchers stated that they had not known anything else.

> Fiona: *I don't feel it's got any disadvantages. You have got your scope for promoting independence as well.*

Table 6.5: Perceptions of the relationship between the RLT model and the action research study.

Informant	How did you make the links with Roper's model?
Day sister	Reinforced a lot and was very useful but that's because of the nursing module I completed (for the diploma in nursing) during the study. We are promoting optimum independence and appropriately using the activities of living. I think sometimes people are too critical of Roper, because I actually find that it works here reasonably well.
Hannah	I haven't got the faintest idea! Something to do with optimum independence.
Fiona	Yes, it was basically promoting independence. There's a framework, and you adapt it to every patient.
Benita	Promoting independence.
Lorraine	I didn't, am I missing something?
Caroline	Linked to personal worries. Yes, we added that a few years ago to the activities of living.
Denise	I don't think I did ... Well, the innovations certainly promoted independence.
Esther	I suppose you are trying to keep the patients independent. You are getting them to medicate themselves, control their pain, more information about their operation and drugs.
Geraldine	I can't really think.

Robinson (1990) believes that a nursing model is not a particularly useful tool as a catalyst for change, and Lister (1991) argues that the RLT model, although potentially useful, allows nurses to maintain their practice and the status quo against many pressures within and outside the profession.

> Its adoption [the RLT model] will not necessarily, and does not in fact, give to nurses a new perspective on nursing activity, or challenge entrenched viewpoints ... it does not necessarily empower nurses to act with their own authority in the patients' interests. (Lister 1991, 210)

The criticisms should be examined alongside how the RLT model was implemented in clinical practice. The model was initially imposed on staff in many clinical areas. Nurses are at different levels of attainment and the models at different stages of clinical and theoretical development. Indeed, if nursing models are considered appropriate, the way in which they are applied in practice may certainly be different for differing specialities.

This study has demonstrated how a nursing model can be utilised as a catalyst for change, how it has enabled practitioners to question the status quo and empowered nurses within a bureaucratic setting.

Meaningful outcomes of the study

Traditionally, outcome studies within the NHS have been almost exclusively concerned with classification and measurement. Patton (1990), however, asserts that when determining outcomes there is a need to identify the importance of the unique meaning of the experience for each person and an overview of the patterns of outcomes.

Outcomes of nurse-led change and development through a critical action research methodology have been identified. Outcomes have been described for patients, co-researchers, managers, myself as an action researcher, the clinical area and the organisation (NHS Trust), see table 6.6. Within an action research study the process and outcomes may be similar or the same. For example, the co-researchers spoke of feelings of empowerment both during the process of innovation implementation and as an outcome of the change process.

Moving forward

Nurse-led change and development was undertaken over a fifteen-month period and reinforced for me the democratic and equitable process of critical action research. The co-researchers chose to participate in the study and identified the innovations, and each felt that their contribution was valued and worthwhile. The study enhanced our professional working lives. We collectively responded to the challenges and positive feedback regarding the three innovations provided by the patients and healthcare colleagues. The ward team became more cohesive, and there was evidence of increased motivation by the co-researchers for further learning and practice development. I had felt equally valued, challenged and enlightened throughout the process. These collective and individual outcomes reinforced for me the significance of the methodology that, as Stringer (1996, 10) states, 'operates

Table 6.6: Outcomes of the action research study for patients, co-researchers, nurse unit manager, action researcher, clinical area and hospital trust.

Patients	Nurses (co-researchers)	Nurse unit manager	Action researcher	Clinical area	Hospital trust
increased psychological and physical independence	more insight into nursing - more questioning of the status quo	eye opener	realisation of personal ideals: learning in clinical practice, shared knowledge, patient participation, nurse empowerment	enhanced team cohesion	resource area for other units
feeling in control	work collaboratively	recognition of nurses' abilities	work collaboratively	group goal attainment	published information booklets
increased knowledge	enhanced knowledge	valuing nurses' ideas	group reflection skills	proactive innovative setting	enhanced patient satisfaction
felt nurses trusted them	enhanced teaching skills	Empowering nurses	insight into strengthening multi-professional collaboration	motivated nurses	enhanced quality of care
reduced feelings of anxiety	feelings of personal achievement		enhanced knowledge	enhanced quality of care	improved staff morale
	enhanced nurse–patient communication				
	increased self-confidence				
	motivated towards further study				
	feeling able to make changes				
	increased writing skills				

at the intellectual level as well as at social, cultural, political, and emotional levels'.

I could certainly move forward and engage in further nurse-led change and development and, indeed, so could the ward team:

Day sister: (evaluation interview) *I think it has done us a lot of good. I really mean that. I think it has given us all something to work towards. We have all seen that we can achieve something. It has put the words 'action research' into perspective, because nobody actually knew what it actually was, and now we are thinking: 'What are we going to do next?'*

Chapter 7
Development of the second study

'I remain firmly committed to action research as a potentially fruitful way to introduce and evaluate innovation in nursing.' (Webb 1993, 131)

Linking factors from the first study

Each action research study is unique and follows its own pattern of development as it emerges in collaboration with participants, in the reality of practice (Meyer 1995). Indeed, the positivist term 'generalisability of findings' is limited (Hart and Bond 1995a), irrelevant (Hendry and Farley 1996, Stringer 1996) and impossible (McKernan 1996). Yet transferable knowledge gleaned from the first study supported by an ongoing critique of the literature should enable a more informed approach to the development of the second action research study.

From the first study, the likelihood of a successful action research study was enhanced by continuous management support, a known and credible facilitator, endorsement of the change by patients and the multi-professional team, a knowledge of the change process, a commitment to shared group reflection and learning, and the implementation of the critical approach to action research. These criteria informed the second study. However, I expected other factors to arise as I was exploring a different context as well as adopting the role of 'outsider' and therefore was not a known or credible facilitator. The past experience of the ethics committee and initial management rejection also necessitated a different approach to these elements of the second study.

Further reflection and analysis of the data from the first study enabled me to gain added insight into the management perspective. Key themes that emerged for the nurse unit manager (NUM) were those of ongoing support, relinquishing control, conflicting loyalties, identifying positive outcomes, enhanced value and respect for staff and an enhanced personal knowledge. While each study is unique, I anticipated that these themes could be useful to explore with managers in the negotiation process of the second study.

The ongoing support for the first study by the NUM was a key strategy for change. From our negotiated agreement, she ensured protected time and ward cover to enable the co-researchers to be released for the planning/problem-solving/evaluation meetings. The NUM provided ongoing interest and positive feedback to the co-researchers. For example, during the three-month pilot study for patient-controlled analgesia (PCA), she reported that one of the consultants thought it was 'the best thing since sliced bread and that all his patients were going to have it'. Legitimation of the innovation by both the NUM and a senior member of the medical staff provided a strong driving force for change.

The NUM's enlightened form of leadership could be viewed as the antithesis to the current culture found within some NHS Trusts. Andrews-Evans (1997) refers to the impossible task for some nurses who are striving to ensure high standards of clinically effective care. Many changes have been imposed on staff, sometimes without clear explanation or the opportunity to advise on the change. For nurses, personal and professional values regarding patient care are often challenged when coping with the demands of working in a bureaucratic organisation. Indeed, by engaging in critical action research we could have been labelled as reprobates, as, according to Coghlan and Brannick (2001), the process might be considered subversive and threatening to existing organisational norms. This is what happened in the second study. As the action researcher I once again, in Coghlan and Brannick's (2001) terms, attempted to generate valid and useful information in order to facilitate free and informed choice in accordance with the theory and practice of critical action research. However, what constituted valid information was equally intensely political.

Consolidating previous knowledge

The outcomes of the first study reflect the nature of post-positivist research, which, for Reason and Marshall (1987), encompasses three perspectives:

1. For them - research makes a contribution to the fund of knowledge.
2. For us - research is a co-operative endeavour that enables us to act effectively in our world.
3. For me - research makes a contribution to my personal development.

I hoped and felt that each of the three perspectives had been achieved. The first perspective - the fund of knowledge derived from the study - demonstrated both deductive and inductive processes. The deductive research process included the application to practice of concepts particularly within the Roper et al. (1990) model, critical social theory, reflective theory, experiential theory and change theory. Inductively derived knowledge emerged, for example, from the co-researchers' reflections on the action research process. This knowledge contributed to the outcome of patient-centred enhancement, which included making time for explanations, treating people as individuals, trusting patients, better patient assessments, non-discrimination and better rapport.

The second perspective of Reason and Marshall (1987) is reflected in our collective ability to challenge and change the status quo for the enhancement of patient care within a bureaucratic setting. We also gained insight and confidence into the complexities of the change process for initiating future practice developments.

The least effective stage of the study was the lack of co-operation from some of the anaesthetists regarding the provision of PCA (page 119). Patients were at risk of harm through the delays that occurred. Feedback avoidance by the co-researchers was also elicited as an ineffective coping strategy for collaborative change.

I am hopeful that experienced nurses, particularly those working in practice development and those with a hospital or community link, will consider adopting the role of critical action research facilitator. There has also been a growing recognition of the potential of the nurse researcher, who is familiar with a setting, to make an active contribution to quality nursing practice (Hanson 1994). Also being recognised is the changing role of nurse educators as important change agents (Walsh 1998), as well as their central role in the process of empowerment (Holloway and Race 1993).

Within the first study I was able to combine the roles of nurse researcher, educator, change agent and, as Holloway and Race (1993, 263) predict, 'assume a collaborative role with practitioners to engage in action research in order to develop the theoretical basis for nursing practice, contribute to the solution of practical problems and enhance the quality of care delivered to patients'. In my role as (clinical link) lecturer I could clearly recognise the importance of integrating knowledge of research, education and change to enhance patient care. I could equally recognise the skills that transfer from the educational to the clinical setting, especially when facilitating life-long adult learning. The study also reinforces the problems as well as the possibilities of working effectively as a researcher, educator and change agent within a dynamic and stressful environment. As Walsh observes:

> It is from within the team that the drive to change must be developed. Bellman (1996) offers a good example of this approach utilising the Roper model ... This is a good example of how the basic philosophy underlying a model can be a catalyst for change ... Alas, this is a single study only ... Nursing will not be able to advance its thinking about nursing unless ideas can be tried out in practice and evaluated. (1998, 132)

The third perspective - undertaking post-positivist research - has not only made a contribution to my personal development; it continues to influence my life. It has confirmed my belief in advancing practice knowledge with practitioners, patients and healthcare workers. The process enabled me to appreciate more clearly the diverse demands on each nurse, which encompassed professional practice and organisational needs. I developed greater insight into the co-researchers' vulnerability, especially regarding writing skills and relationships with medical staff. Yet the study had contributed to their personal and professional development. Another rewarding aspect of the study was undertaking patient interviews and feeding back their responses to the co-researchers. Many patients are at their most vulnerable while in hospital. I felt a sense of achievement to have moved them beyond the 'all the nurses here are wonderful' stage (a common response, especially in older patients) to elicit more meaningful perspectives.

In preparation for the second action research study and throughout the research process, I clearly identified similarities and differences between the two studies. These comparisons are perceived as significant and consequently are discussed within this and the following chapters.

Objectives of the second study

Nurse-led change and development in the second action research study was undertaken in a day surgery unit (DSU). One of the most profound changes in modern times to have affected surgical nursing and acute care in general has been the growing number of patients undergoing day surgery (Audit Commission 1990). The starting point for the second study was from previous nursing research that had explored the experience of day surgery patients. To ensure anonymity for the DSU the author of this research will not be identified. One of the key recommendations was to initiate an action research study to explore and resolve day surgery patient-specific problems. The focus for change therefore became the creation of an appropriate environment for paediatric care, as identified by the DSU co-researchers.

The study attempted to empower day surgery staff to initiate, action plan, implement and evaluate a change strategy (primarily) regarding paediatric provision. The three key objectives were:

- to explore the perceptions of day surgery staff, patients and carers, regarding paediatric provision
- to identify factors associated with challenging and changing the status quo
- to investigate the process and outcomes from group reflection on changing practice

Data collection methods

A major strength of action research is the opportunity to use many different sources of evidence in an effort to develop converging lines of enquiry, sometimes termed 'triangulation' (Hugentobler et al. 1992). Indeed, Jones (1996) uses triangulation in clinical practice for a greater understanding of a wider range of phenomena, participants, perspectives, experiences and activities under investigation. (For a discussion of triangulation see the section 'Triangulation of data' in chapter 4.) I gained confidence from the first study in the use of the micro-cassette for taping group discussions and interviews, in writing personal journal reflections and in making field notes. I chose, therefore, to utilise these methods for the second study. I also drew on my experience in the first study to facilitate the development of the DSU staff and patient questionnaires. This multimethod approach enabled me to gain increased understanding of the nature of the identified problems and the process and outcomes of change.

I maintained a journal for my personal reflections, which I recorded after each group meeting. Reflective insights that occurred at random were captured on any available scrap of paper and then transferred to the journal as soon as possible. To lessen anxiety and potential intimidation, descriptive field notes replaced the micro-cassette at the first meeting with the theatre manager, with the co-researchers (at our fortnightly meetings) and at the DSU nursing staff feedback session (towards the end of the study). I also had to resort to field notes when, on one occasion, there was a fault with the micro-cassette. The stages and process of the second action research study are delineated in table 7.1.

Table 7.1: The stages and process of the second action research study.

STAGES	PROCESS
1. **Initiating the study**	* negotiated agreements with managers * ethics committee * selection of co-researchers * field notes

2. **Problem identification**
  a) need to improve the quality of care for children
  b) need to improve drinks facility for staff/patients
	* group meetings (3)
	* audiotaped group discussion
	* reflection-on-action
	* field notes/personal journal reflections
	* staff feedback
	* literature sources

3. **Planning** a) quality of care for children	* audiotaped group meetings (5) * stakeholders' views * development/piloting of questionnaires (80) * audit department & management input * field notes/personal journal reflections
b) drinks provision	* audiotaped group discussion * stakeholders' views * personal journal reflections
4. **Implementation** a) quality of care for children	* co-researcher strategy * co-researcher journals * collaborative analysis
b) drinks provision	* co-researcher strategy
5. **Process evaluation**	* audiotaped group meeting * audiotaped group interview * nursing staff feedback meeting * field notes/personal journal reflections * theatre manager interview * NHS Trust interim report * action researcher reflexivity

The setting

The second study was undertaken in a purpose-built DSU, situated within the grounds of a district general hospital. The DSU replaced a smaller DSU, which was originally sited at a recently closed NHS Trust hospital a few miles away. Some of the staff had transferred from the unit to the new DSU.

The DSU consisted of a reception area, a small, quieter reception area (for ophthalmic patients), a small children's play room, two consulting rooms, four operating theatres, a pre- and post-operative open plan area with space for 24 trolleys plus four individual rooms and a staff lounge. Patients were admitted from the age of one. Surgery/treatments performed include herniorrhaphy, laparoscopic cholecystectomy, removal of breast lumps, stripping of varicose veins, cataract removal, circumcision, termination of pregnancy, ear, nose and throat surgery, etc.

The DSU had been opened eight months when the study commenced. The staff included a DSU manager (G grade) who reported to a newly appointed theatre manager (H grade). The DSU manager was working her notice prior to retirement. A new DSU manager had yet to be appointed. The number of nursing and health-care support staff in the DSU is listed in table 7.2. Of the staff nurses there were five F grade, 17 E grade (one male), four D grade and eight worked full time. There were six enrolled nurses, one of whom worked full-time. The remainder of the nursing and support staff included four healthcare assistants (one full-time), six bank nursing staff, five operating department personnel (three full-time) plus one trainee. The medical staff to the unit included 25 surgeons (five female) and 11 anaesthetists (two female). The director of the DSU was a female consultant anaesthetist. There were seven clerical staff and one porter. No student nurses accessed the DSU at that time.

DSU staff

Table 7.2: The 91 staff of the DSU.

Registered nurses (including DSU manager)	26 (18 part-time)
Enrolled nurses	6 (5 part- time)
Healthcare assistants	4 (2 part-time)
Operating department personnel	5 + 1trainee (2 part-time)
Surgeons	25
Anaesthetists	11
Clerical staff	7
Porter	1
Bank nursing staff	6

The nursing staff were able to gain experience in all areas of the DSU. There was a system of rotation which encompassed time spent in pre-admission and pre-operative preparation, theatre experience, post-operative recovery and discharge provision. According to Morgan and Reynolds (1991), a system of rotation was seen by nurses to enhance their job satisfaction. It made the work more interesting, contributed to better staff relationships and improved the quality of patient care by enabling the nursing staff to have a greater understanding of the whole of the patient's experience. However, this was also seen as a potential problem as it could necessitate extensive in-service training.

Service provision in the DSU reflected surgeons' operating times, which were, in the main, fixed to specific days with either morning or afternoon sessions. Adults and children were seen in the pre-admission clinic and admitted together. The majority of patients returned home the same day, having received both verbal and written information regarding rehabilitation. On rare occasions, a patient may have been admitted to the main hospital for further observation. A follow-up telephone call was made by a nurse to all DSU patients within 24 hours of discharge. The DSU was operational on five days a week, but, during the study, there were ongoing discussions regarding the viability of Saturday opening.

Development of the study

The study was commenced as a result of previous research undertaken by a lecturer in nursing. Her research, an exploration of the lived experience of DSU patients, was undertaken in the now closed DSU. A number of the staff at the new centre, including two of the co-researchers, had known of the lecturer's (unpublished) work. The aim of the study was to describe the experiences of people as they contemplate, undergo and recover from day surgery.

The research enabled the researcher/lecturer, an experienced surgical nurse, to elicit assumptions and preconceptions from eight patients undergoing hernia repair. Three interviews were undertaken with each participant one to two weeks prior to surgery, on the morning or afternoon of surgery and two weeks following surgery. The analysis, using Colaizzi's (1978) framework, demonstrated the complexity of contemplating, undergoing and recovering from day surgery. Recommendations included the need to explore the lived experiences of relatives/carers of day surgery patients who, it was discovered, were more fearful and anxious than the patients. A recurring theme was the need for greater information exchange between patient and healthcare professional with a proposal to consider the creation of a pre-admission clinic. An action research project was recommended to implement and evaluate this proposal.

While acknowledging the need for the study and the opportunity to participate in another change process, I felt quite apprehensive at the thought of being an unknown 'outsider'. Prior to embarking on the study, I contacted the lecturer/researcher for some 'insider' information particularly regarding her perceptions of the organisational culture. She suggested that she attend the first introductory meeting in the DSU; this was most supportive. She also expressed a desire to participate as a co-researcher. Unfortunately, when the time came, she could do neither, owing to increasing demands on her time within the university.

From my experience in the first study, I needed initially both to explore the action research approach and to seek permission from the director of patient services. In the first study my attempt to gain permission to undertake the study had initially resulted in failure. This time I telephoned rather than wrote to the director. She was supportive of nursing research and most receptive to the study. No formal contract was considered necessary. The agreement is described in my journal as 'professional good will'. A follow-up letter confirmed our arrangement. My enthusiasm to proceed had to be constrained for two reasons. I was unable to commence the study until the newly appointed theatre manager had finished her period of orientation, and I needed to obtain ethical clearance.

A positive outcome had resulted from speaking directly to the director; I chose the same approach for the ethics committee. I telephoned the secretary of the ethics committee to inquire whether there was a need to complete the traditional research approval form. I explained that from past experience the format was inappropriate as it was primarily for the randomised control trial with just one page for qualitative research. I offered instead to submit an outline of the action research approach and the proposed study. Unlike the first study where I followed the normal channels, this approach resulted in a successful outcome at the first attempt.

My initial meeting with the new theatre manager (TM) seemed hopeful (journal note). Yet she made it clear that she had little choice but to agree to the study. At that time she had not yet met with the DSU staff. As she was new to the organisation, she could not provide me with any detailed insights into the DSU, for example the extent to which nursing research was applied in practice, the management, education and clinical practice support for nursing staff, innovation in practice or collaborative multi-professional relationships. She stated that the hospital was currently undertaking a major internal reorganisation. Her initial impressions were that many of the nurses were very experienced but had not updated their knowledge, or had not been encouraged to update, and that little in-service education appeared to exist.

The action research approach appeared interesting to the TM as her previous experience was of top-down management initiatives. I provided detailed information regarding the process of the first study, and her initial reaction was, '*Sounds exciting!*' (field note). I stressed the importance of support and participation from the DSU manager. It was then that I was informed that the present manager was about to retire. Her replacement was yet to be appointed. The post was about to be readvertised as no suitable applicant had initially applied.

I explained that, while in the first study I was able to engage with all the staff, this would not appear to be feasible in a unit with at least 30 nursing staff. A different strategy would have to be adopted. I left the TM with a copy of the article 'Action Research' (Webb 1996), an updated version of the handout used in the first study. Her follow-up telephone call confirmed her commitment to the study. With some reservation, I agreed that she would introduce the study at her first meeting with all the DSU staff, select the co-researchers, provide each co-researcher with an updated copy of the Webb (1996) article and introduce me to the co-researchers at our first meeting.

I could recognise the TM's need to establish a power-base, but I felt that the study would be perceived to be 'top-down'. I was also concerned about the need for accurate information to ensure informed consent and also needed reassurance regarding the verbal commitment to 'protected time' for the co-researchers. Bartunek and Louis (1996) recognise that informed consent in joint insider/outsider studies is problematic. As neither the action researcher nor the co-researchers will have full knowledge of the events that will unfold during the study, the authors suggest that a revised form of informed consent seems warranted. They suggest that consent is not something that can be handled once and for all at the beginning of the study; consent is (re)negotiated at different points in the research cycle.

My fears were allayed at the first meeting, four weeks later, when I was able to explore the information given to the co-researchers and agree the nature of informed consent. A fortnightly one-hour meeting was negotiated with the retiring DSU manager. In all, eight of the nine meetings were audiotaped.

Selection of co-researchers

I had agreed to the selection of the co-researchers by their senior manager but had anxieties regarding my powerlessness in the process. I hoped the TM would adopt a democratic process of co-researcher self-selection. I also reflected on whether I could facilitate an action research study with strangers. I could not assess, even intuitively, their motivation, commitment and abilities. Yet I believe that all healthcare staff should be enabled to participate in change. We would all be participating in a developmental process with, hopefully, quality outcomes. I could meet the challenge knowing that I had management support. However it would be important to reinforce the managerial commitment and, as in the first study (with the NUM), I would ensure that I communicated with the TM on a regular basis.

Four staff were initially to participate in the study. I hoped that they were staff members who were respected by their peers and had a good working relationship with the DSU manager. They may also have been considered informal leaders within the DSU. Although the four members of staff did not volunteer, as recommended by Carr and Kemmis (1986), they agreed to participate. The criteria for choosing the 'action researcher outsider' include establishing trust, the ability to work jointly and their research skill (Bartunek and Louis 1996, p. 25). Although they had not chosen me, I hoped that I could fulfil these essential criteria.

The fifth co-researcher, Nina, the part-time nurse lecturer to the DSU, approached me in the corridor at the end of the first co-researcher meeting. She asked if she could participate as she felt that the action research study was a positive move, especially in the current political climate. Her view on the bottom-up approach to change was enlightening:

> Nina: *Surely it's the only thing left that you can do for them now!* (field note)

Within the new DSU her initial attempts at creating a shared learning culture had not been well supported. She currently felt frustrated in her role but was hopeful that the new TM and DSU managers would value her input. The five co-researchers were:

Rebecca	E-grade staff nurse (part-time)
Jenny	E-grade staff nurse (full-time)
Patsy	Healthcare assistant (part-time)
Chris	Operating department assistant (part-time)
Nina	Nurse lecturer (part-time)

Rebecca and Chris were redeployed from the recently closed DSU. At the commencement of the study, Nina had just submitted her dissertation for the award of MSc in Health Studies. Rebecca and Jenny were registered general nurses; no other formal education courses had been undertaken. Patsy and Chris had received only on-site training. I wondered, as Morgan and Reynolds (1991) highlight, whether working in day surgery was seen to be limiting for career prospects. Yet the authors also identified a stable core of nurses who 'stay for long periods and find the work convenient and satisfying' (Morgan and Reynolds 1991, 71).

Preparations

A priority for me was to establish effective open communication with both the retiring DSU manager and her replacement, who were working together through the transition period. I emphasised to both my role as a research facilitator, trying to establish collaborative practice and engagement with all staff. I wanted the process to be seen as non-threatening, to benefit both patients and staff and explained that the co-researchers and I very much hoped that the newly appointed DSU (and the out-going) manager would participate in the process. Unfortunately, neither of them ever did. I stated (as in the first study) that patient care, rather than the meetings, would be the priority. For example, even with agreed 'protected time' on occasions staff sickness might necessitate a co-researcher replacing one of her colleagues (and foregoing a meeting). The meetings would be kept to time. After each fortnightly meeting with the co-researchers I fed back to the DSU manager both verbally (whenever possible) and, on three occasions, in writing. I wanted to inform her of progress and to try to elicit her support over time. The same information was also forwarded to the TM.

There was no purpose-built seminar room or designated teaching area within the whole of the newly built DSU; so every fortnight, prior to each group meeting, I had to renegotiate with the DSU manager a site for the meeting. The first meeting with the co-researchers took place in the children's small play room (no children were present at the time!). At the first meeting the TM introduced me to the four co-researchers (the fifth co-researcher, Nina, would join us at the next meeting). The TM stated her commitment to the study.

As an unknown outsider I knew that one of my key aims was to develop a trusting relationship over time with the co-researchers (and the DSU manager). I explained the nature of the study, my role as facilitator/researcher and discussed the process and outcomes of the first action research study. The co-researchers were extremely interested in the first study; this also helped to establish my credibility as I could demonstrate that I appreciated the demands of surgical nursing practice. I introduced the co-researchers to the micro-cassette, which, with expressions of good-humoured disdain, they agreed could be used from the second meeting onwards. None of the co-researchers at that time had read the action research article, Webb 1996, that the TM had provided, on my suggestion, the month before. I explored their initial understanding of the study and the nature of informed consent. I wanted them to have as much information as possible to enable a reasoned judgement prior to signing the consent form. I followed Williams' (1995) advice to view informed consent as a continuous process where it is made clear at the outset to participants that I did not know the exact and precise progression of the research. Each co-researcher agreed to sign the consent form to participate.

An assumption of mine that was soon dispelled was that the co-researchers knew one another and had worked together. This revelation occurred during our initial introductions. Although they were all employed as the DSU opened, eight months prior to the study, two of the co-researchers had never met, not even in the staff lounge! The fact that I was not the only stranger present at the first meeting did not appear to present a problem.

The co-researchers shared their knowledge and perceptions of the unit with one another and started to identify current issues. I shared one of the significant problems that the lecturer/researcher had identified from her study - there was a need for an intermediate meeting point for patients and healthcare staff which should occur between being seen in outpatients and the day of surgery, i.e. establish a pre-admission clinic.

> Rebecca: *We do now have a pre-admission clinic, but we could do with one just for children.*

This insight generated much discussion, possibly reinforced by our environment. We were seated on low-slung chairs surrounded by toys, children's books, crayons and posters. Chris moved the suggestion one stage further and raised the possibility of a dedicated day in the DSU just for paediatric surgery. She felt that this would address some of the problems that she and her colleagues were experiencing. A specified day for children had been the norm at the now closed DSU, where both she and Rebecca had previously worked. They had valued the opportunity to focus specifically on children and their carers and believed that this promoted safer working practices. The meeting concluded with a commitment to reflect on this proposal as well as any other significant issues and to start to elicit colleagues' views on the need for change. In my journal I reflected on the speed at which a key issue had been identified, but this had also occurred in the first study. The group had highlighted a patient-focused change that, if considered feasible, would have major implications for every staff member in the DSU.

Moving forward

Compared to the preparation for the first action research study, the initial arrangements for this study were completed with relative ease. As an outsider I had obtained support from the ethics committee, the director and theatre manager without any real difficulty. I had engaged with the co-researchers, who appeared motivated and had started to share their values regarding day-surgery nursing. Yet I had two underlying anxieties. I could only hope that a newly appointed DSU manager would support the initiative and eventually become a coresearcher. Also, the staff of the DSU were already experiencing two major changes: the loss of two managers in short succession and an overall management reorganisation. Would the action research study survive in the midst of major organisational change? I hoped that it would confirm my previous argument:

> Initiating an action research study in the midst of political and organisational change provides an open format for group discussion and support and enables the powerless group to become proactive by initiating their own agenda for change. (Bellman 1996, 133)

Chapter 8
Advancing the change process

> 'Our ultimate goal is to provide a context that enables diverse stakeholders to work collaboratively toward solutions to the significant problems that confront them.' (Stringer 1999)

Unfreezing is the first of three steps of the change process, as described by Lewin (1952). During this phase, participants recognise the need for a change, work to diagnose the problem and generate a solution by selecting from a number of alternative approaches.

Identifying a key problem

A consensus on exploring the need to have a dedicated day for children was agreed at the second meeting with all five of the co-researchers present. They had been exploring their colleagues' views:

> Loretta: *So I remember, Rebecca, you were talking about having a specific day or half a day for children.*
> Rebecca: *A lot of people are in favour of that.*

Reflections on practice were shared by Jenny, which reinforced the need for a specific day. It would provide enhanced care for the child as well as support for the nurse:

> *I have just had a child I could not control, and I am not paediatric trained. He was a nightmare that child, hit everybody; I couldn't do a thing with him. I also had another child who I was told could go 'flat', because she had had Pethidine. Three others grizzling. I was at the point where I wanted to go in the corner and grizzle*

177

> *myself. We have two paediatric trained nurses but neither were on duty. If we had a paediatric day, then you would make sure that they were on duty. They could be the leaders of the team that day.*

Chris identified that a dedicated day would also promote safer working practices in the operating theatre:

> *I know from our end* [in the operating theatre] *we would prefer to have just a list of paeds; then we'd all know where we are and what we are doing, because quite often we don't know that there are paeds on the list until we actually get it. If you don't look at the age, they don't have to put the age on the list, just the date of birth and even then you are mainly thinking 'adults'. You prepare the instruments and, golly, can't use those - they are too big. With a paediatric day we would have all the proper equipment prepared right at the start.*

We explored different strategies to obtain all the stakeholders' views. Ideas generated included my attendance at the next nursing staff meeting, noting patients' views, asking clerical staff, devising a questionnaire for both staff and patients and:

> Rebecca: *What if we picked the surgeons' brains and had a word with them to see how they felt about it?*

The co-researchers felt that this may be an opportune time to review paediatric provision, especially with a new DSU manager in place:

> Jenny: *I think if A. was going to remain in charge we wouldn't get a paediatrics day, because this subject has been broached before, but with B. we might have a bit more success.*
> Rebecca: *I don't know why A. is resisting ... Oh I think she said something along the lines of 'I'm not having 24 trolleys with screaming children!'*

However, the co-researchers perceived the surgeons as potentially the main group to resist change. It was hoped that problems could be resolved:

> Chris: *I don't see why surgeons can't transfer paediatrics to other surgeons' lists if they know there is going to be a paediatric day or half a day or whatever. They could be transferred to that surgeon that likes doing paediatrics. End of problem!*

Positive reflections on past experiences were shared by Chris and Rebecca; a rosy picture was painted. Yet the comments appeared to be an accurate account of recent experience not distorted by time. They were 'legitimised' by the Clinical Director of the DSU (a consultant anaesthetist) who attended one of the meetings:

> *What I would like is a first-class service for everybody, that is the optimum and that is how we ran it when we had it at X. hospital ... I am certainly very keen to have a day's work with just paediatric surgery.*

She also commented on the staff's and patients' perspectives:

> *I know that the recovery area was quite a worry for V. She doesn't like having children in there with adults, and I know that some adults have refused to go into recovery when there have been children in there, so it is a bit of a problem.*

Other problems

Also at the second meeting another problem was raised by Patsy:

> *One of the girls has said we need a vending machine for staff and patients. I did bring this up at a staff meeting some time ago. Relatives are often here all day, especially parents who don't want to leave the unit. We get so thirsty, even a machine where we could get cold water. A proper vending machine even ... we can't get out, we have half an hour lunchbreak, and if we have forgotten to bring our lunch.*
> Loretta: *So who was supposed to take some action on the vending machine?*
> Patsy: *Well, A.* [retiring DSU manager] *said she was going to, but we haven't actually had anything.*
> Jenny: *They have got those vending machines at Z*

> *hospital* [part of the trust] *to get sandwiches and crisps. We will have a word with B* [newly appointed DSU manager]. *Yes, I don't see why we shouldn't.*

Other problems were also aired which enabled the co-researchers to get things off their chest and enabled me to glean more insight into the culture of the DSU and the organisation. For example, the organisational policy for general supplies had been recently changed but when put into action had resulted in increased stress for the co-researchers and a reduced service to patients:

> Chris: *When the nurses did their own ordering, then you knew what you wanted ... but this girl that comes from supplies hasn't got a clue, because she is not familiar with surgery. We have loads of glove sizes that we don't want and not enough of the glove sizes that we do want. It is the same with sutures - we are getting loads of sutures that we don't need and not enough of the sutures that we do need. You can't seem to get through to them they are not supplying what we need.*
> Loretta: *Who decides how many you want in the first place?*
> Chris: *It's agreed with the manager. Obviously, if it's not enough, you can go back and change it.*
> Patsy: *The girl went away for two weeks on holiday and didn't ask somebody to take it on for the two weeks that she was on holiday so then we had no top-up supplies for two weeks.*

Presenting these issues at the next DSU nursing staff meeting seemed a very relevant suggestion. It would also be an opportunity to engage with the other DSU nursing staff. I could clarify the study and hope to engender interest and involvement.

> Loretta: *Can I get a feel for the meetings that you have? Don't look at me like that!* [laughter]
> Rebecca: *I just thought the last one was a waste of time. I just thought I can't believe that this is meant to be a two-way process ... because we wanted to bring up about this project, to let people know so that they could come back to us, but we didn't have a chance.*

Unfortunately, work commitments prevented me from attending. At the end of the second co-researcher meeting I recapped on our discussions and our action plan. I felt that there was a commitment to pursue paediatric provision. Jenny, an experienced nurse and mother, had revealed that she lacked the confidence and knowledge to care for children within the DSU environment. This was especially as she had not had paediatric nurse support. The co-researchers agreed. How many other staff members felt the same? Of the other issues raised, the co-researchers decided to pursue the vending machine. Patsy volunteered to oversee the vending machine project. The co-researchers asked me to confront the DSU managers regarding all the problems. Disempowering language and feelings of disillusionment were apparent; this was now evidenced by feedback avoidance (which was also evident in the first study, see page 107). However, in the first study this issue related to medical staff. These co-researchers seemed reluctant to feed back to their nurse managers.

> Jenny: *If you sound A. and B. [DSU managers] out.*
> Loretta: *You want me to do it?*
> Jenny: *I thought you were offering to do it.*
> Loretta: *Well, if that's what you want.*
> Rebecca: *I think we ought to do it. I think it should come from us really honestly and truthfully.*
> Loretta: *I think that would be the best idea ... I will reinforce the issues. It would be a nice move on B.'s part to implement a vending machine very soon after she arrives, a very popular move, wouldn't it?*
> Nina: *It would be very popular.*

It was also agreed that before the next meeting Nina (lecturer) and I would explore the day-surgery literature regarding paediatric provision. Evidence from the literature should support the proposed innovation.

Supporting evidence from the literature

The literature regarding day surgery clearly supported the need for a change in the quality of paediatric care provision in the DSU. The evidence enlightened us; it enabled us to more fully appreciate the significance of the proposed innovation and it enhanced our motivation for change. The literature encompassed government documents, national and professional organisational reports and day-surgery journal articles. Statistics from the Department of Health (1997) revealed that on average 60% of patients from waiting lists were treated as day cases in 1996/97. In relation to paediatrics, the Royal College of Surgeons (1992) estimate that probably 50% of all surgical procedures required in infancy and childhood could be performed on a day-case basis; of these some 60% would be under five years of age.

It was an overwhelming experience for us all to discover that the advantages of a day unit specifically for children were identified many years ago in the early 1970s (Atwell et al. 1997). The advantages proposed by the authors encompass current initiatives within the NHS and include:

- reduced psychological disturbance for the child and carer (quality of care)
- a reduction in inpatient beds and the integration of hospital and community services (care in the community)
- the cost-effectiveness of the change (health economics)
- a reduction in waiting-list time (Patient's Charter) and reduced cross infection (risk management)

These criteria for change reflect the need for special arrangements for children as proposed by the Audit Commission's (1990) operational policy for DSUs.

The following year the Department of Health, supported by the organisation, Caring for Children in the Health Services (CCHS 1991), introduced twelve standards of care for paediatric provision (see table 8.1). Although there has been repeated support for the twelve quality standards (Thornes 1991, Morton 1993, Leenders 1996), they are often not implemented, owing to the lack of attention to the special needs of children and their families by many clinicians, managers and other staff (Nuffield Hospitals 1994, Leenders 1996). The standards have been incorporated into the King's Fund's (1991) Core Standards for Clinical Services Audit Tool.

The standards (table 8.1) that the co-researchers felt were currently implemented in the DSU were numbers 2, 4, 6, 8, 9, 11, 12 ; number 10 needed improvement. They found it difficult to comprehend why the other standards had not been addressed, i.e. numbers 1, 3, 5 and, in particular, number 7. This standard requires nurses, anaesthetists and surgeons to be trained in the care of children. The Royal College of Surgeons (1992) recognises the need for paediatric anaesthetists and nurses in day surgery, but there is no reference to the need for surgeons with paediatric expertise. Thornes (1991) criticises surgeons who have difficulty in altering their long-standing methods, habits and attitudes regarding the care of children. In particular she was critical of surgeons

Table 8.1: The twelve paediatric quality standards (CCHS 1991).

TWELVE QUALITY STANDARDS

A planned package of care for day-care admission

1. The admission is planned in an **integrated** way to include **pre-admission,** day-of-admission and post-admission care, and to incorporate the concept of a planned transfer of care to primary and/or community services.
2. The child and parent are offered preparation both before and during the day of admission.
3. Specific written information is provided to ensure that parents understand their responsibilities throughout the episode.
4. The child is admitted to an area designated for day cases and not mixed with acutely ill inpatients.
5. **The child is neither admitted nor treated alongside adults.**
6. The child is cared for by identified staff specifically designated to the day-case area.
7. **Medical, nursing and all other staff are trained for and skilled in work with children and their families, in addition to the expertise needed for day-case work.**
8. The organisation and delivery of patient care are planned specifically for day cases so that every child is likely to be discharged within the day.
9. The building, equipment and furnishings comply with safety standards for children.
10. **The environment is homely and includes areas for play and other activities designed for children and young people.**
11. Essential documentation, including communication with the primary and/or community services, is completed before each child goes home so that after-care and follow-up consultations are not delayed.
12. Once care has been transferred to the home, nursing support is provided, at a doctor's request, by nurses trained in the care of sick children.

who are adult consultants but operate on children. However, there is recognition of the need for a specified day:

> Children should therefore be admitted either to a children's day unit or to a general day unit reserved for children on one day (in the week or month, depending on the workload) ... Skilled anaesthetists and children's nurses must be available. (Royal College of Surgeons, 1992, 11-12)

Exploring the literature reinforced for me a 'policy-reality gap', i.e. the extent to which the information contained in government reports and professional guidelines is actually implemented in practice. With the opening of a new DSU, the co-researchers felt that there had been a missed opportunity. Patterns of work had now become established, which might be difficult to change. They also considered the extent to which the CCHS standards had actually been incorporated into the DSU local audit process (that was undertaken prior to commencement of the study). The importance of auditing day-surgery clinical services has been recognised (Leenders 1996). A quality leadership plan is proposed that identifies both patient care and staff development issues within clinical audit:

> In day surgery we look at improvements by a 'bottom-up approach'. (Carrington 1993, 15)

Indeed, this approach would enable the issue of paediatric standards of care to be addressed.

Within the literature it was also encouraging to find an article that described the adaptation of an adult DSU for paediatric work (Nicholl et al. 1996). The authors advocate a collaborative multi-professional approach to change. Much practical advice was provided and some key areas for consideration are identified in table 8.2.

Table 8.2: Key areas for consideration in the adaptation of an adult DSU for children (Nicholl et al. 1996).

- **Physical modifications** - safety notices, play area with children's pictures and posters, television and video, child toilet seats/small steps/potties
- **Equipment** - paediatric-specific for anaesthesia, surgery, resuscitation and drugs
- **Staffing** - appointment of a registered sick-children's nurse
- **Pre-operative screening and information for parents** - pre-admission clinic and child-specific information leaflets, 'adult information leaflets are not satisfactory for this purpose'
- **Gathering children together** - *'children-only lists are ideal*, allowing part of the DSU to be adapted and function accordingly for that session. At present our ENT surgeons have a monthly paediatric list, while those with a smaller requirement, e.g. orthopaedics, gather children together for occasional sessions on a less frequent basis'

Conclusions

The conclusions from the article reassured us that the cost of adaptation was small and that the physical modifications could be left in place, as they did not affect adult care. Also, careful planning of operating lists only with children meant that they did not mix with adult patients, and this enabled staff to be totally geared to the needs of children.

The information was clearly relevant to our needs, and I offered to telephone this unit to discuss the change process. The nurse manager confirmed that the innovation had been audited with patients/users and staff, with positive outcomes identified for both. There had been few problems as the change had been initially management led with medical and nursing staff recognising a need for change. The unit was smaller than the DSU with fewer surgeons to accommodate. There was an open invitation to contact the unit for ongoing information.

The need for change was also reinforced by the paediatric nursing literature. For example, Thornes states:

> Nurses have a better understanding of children's needs
> than most senior managers and a more detailed knowl-
> edge of what actually happens on the wards than many
> of their medical colleagues. (1991, 14)

This perspective is endorsed by Foale (1991), who challenges certain outdated attitudes that govern paediatric practice. She advocates open discussion and debate of experiences and problems of child care. Yet, in spite of these pleas for changes, the problems remain: 'the physical environment provided for the (paediatric) day-case unit was woefully below the standards identified by the government' (While and Wilcox 1994, 56). Further relevant literature, in the form of a booklet, on the well-being of a child undergoing surgery in the adult peri-operative environment (National Association of Theatre Nurses 1996) was provided by Nina. She also distributed the information to staff of the unit, including the DSU manager. The aim of the booklet was 'to promote and challenge established nursing practice which in turn would enable the development of local protocols to enhance quality paediatric care'. This would appear to be a wholly worthwhile yet rather naïve assumption. I began to reflect on the desirability of a discussion on the complexities of change in all literature that advocates changing clinical practice.

Shared perspectives

The third meeting encompassed initial staff feedback regarding the proposed innovation, as well as the sharing of information from the literature. The informal feedback from the co-researchers reflected the DSU staff's diverse views. I explained that within any change process there will be keen enthusiasts/innovators as well as laggards, early and late adopters, etc. (Rogers 1995). Individuals who were strong resistors to change needed to be identified and their views seriously considered.

> Chris: *Mr S.* [surgeon] *is quite happy about having a paediatric day, but then he always was.*
> Rebecca: *I have spoken to Mr H.* [surgeon] ; *he is not happy. He doesn't really want one ... I couldn't really understand what he was saying. Something about you lose out on your quota and most of the surgery then starts going to P. hospital. I couldn't understand how!*
> Jenny: *I have spoken to one of the staff nurses who is paediatric trained. She had a lot of doubts about it because there isn't a big enough area for the children to play. When I suggested some simple improvements like ... she said she'd never thought about that. You get a different response when you start to explain what we could do if we were allowed.*
> Chris: *I know I keep harping back to X. hospital, but we used to do that. Pictures up, toys all over the place - we were geared up for children. The feedback that we had from parents was absolutely super; they thought it worked really well. The kids were happy, the parents were happy and the staff were happy! The surgeons who worked there that I have spoken to are all for it.*
> Nina: *There should be continuity. I know that in main theatres they are now required to have a dedicated paediatric recovery area.*

None of the co-researchers had broached the topic with parents and patients as they wished to 'sound out' the staff's views first. Patsy shared the staff's enthusiasm for the other identified problem:

> A lot of the staff felt that even a drinks machine rather than a vending machine would be preferable to what there is now - nothing.

Nina and I shared our findings from the day-surgery literature (as discussed on pages 181–185).

> Nina: *There's a wealth of evidence in the literature.*

This undoubtedly reinforced the commitment from the co-researchers to explore the need for change. Values were exchanged:

> Loretta: *All this about empowering patients now is very important. More and more, the patient should be listened to.*
> Jenny: *We should be improving things for the child.*
> Chris: *But then at the end of the day surely their* [DSU staff] *priority should be providing a quality service.*
> Nina: *That's how we see it, but that isn't always how they see it.*

Co-researchers' reading avoidance

After sharing my follow-up telephone call regarding adapting an adult DSU for children (Nicholl et al. 1996), I offered to photocopy the article for everyone. All agreed but said that they (the co-researchers excluding Nina) had not as yet read the first article on action research (Webb 1996), which they had now had for six weeks. It became increasingly apparent throughout the study that suggested reading was not considered important. There were a number of ongoing examples of reading avoidance:

> Loretta: *I sent you a copy of the Royal College of Surgeon's guidelines. I was just delighted when it turned up. Have you read it?*
> Jenny: *I really haven't.*
> Patsy: *I haven't got round to reading it yet.* [general agreement]
> Loretta: *Would you like me to review the important bits?*
> Rebecca: *Yes, would you?*

Two weeks after Nina had distributed the newly published booklet - *Nursing the Paediatric Patient in the Adult Peri-Operative Environment* (National Association of Theatre Nurses 1996):

> Loretta: *Did you have a chance to read it?*
> Rebecca: *To be honest I haven't.* [general agreement]

Preparing the way for paediatric provision

The first three meetings enabled the co-researchers to identify and begin to explore the process of change. The evidence for specific paediatric provision was repeatedly endorsed in the literature. The outcome of informally gauging some of their colleagues' views was to explore further the identified problem. The co-researchers now needed formally to explore the issue with all their peers, medical staff and the DSU manager. Evidence for change from patients was especially important. It was agreed to develop two questionnaires regarding paediatric provision; one would be sent to all staff of the DSU and the other to a selection of adult patients/children/carers. The next five planning meetings involved the development and piloting of questionnaires and the creation of a co-researcher-led implementation strategy.

Questionnaire development

The co-researchers agreed that an analysis of DSU staff and users' questionnaire responses would inform the need to review the current quality of paediatric provision. There was no readily available valid and reliable questionnaire to be found in the literature; so, as in the first study, I facilitated the process of questionnaire development. McKernan (1996) acknowledges this methodological 'eclective-innovative' approach. He states that researchers may have to design new instruments and techniques to gather data, as dictated by the novelty of the problem. He believes that there is no preferred method, although triangulation of methods, perspectives and theories is desirable. As in the first study triangulation was in evidence by the multi-method approaches that were undertaken (see table 7.1, p. 168). The co-researchers' practice knowledge and the day-surgery literature informed the development of the questionnaires (see tables 8.3 and 8.4).

> Loretta: *For question one do I put nurse at the top, then surgeon, anaesthetist, or do I start with porter?*
> Nina: *Alphabetical order!*
> Loretta: *Everything that you have said I could include, like should we have a day dedicated to children? How often do you think it should be: once a week, every fortnight, every six weeks? I could devise something like that, and then I could send it to each of you for comments and to add any further questions.*

Throughout the questionnaire-development meetings, I anticipated that Nina might well challenge the process. She felt justified in doing so as she had used a questionnaire in the research study for her higher degree. She was familiar with the positivist approach to questionnaire

Table 8.3: Development of the DSU staff questionnaire.

STAFF QUESTIONNAIRE - CARE OF CHILDREN	
Question	**Derivative**
1. Please indicate your status.	Co-researchers
2. Should there be a day dedicated to the needs of paediatric patients?	Rebecca and Chris/literature
3. If you believe that there should be a day dedicated specifically for children, how often should this occur?	Co-researchers
4. If you are satisfied with the present arrangement, please say why.	Co-researchers
5. Which day of the week would appear to be the most suitable to be dedicated to children and why?	Co-researchers
6. Which age group do you think is appropriate to attend on this day?	Jenny
7. Should there be a specific paediatric pre-admission clinic	Rebecca, prior research/literature
8. If you agree with no.7, on which day of the week should it be held and why?	Rebecca
9. Is the proportion of paediatric nurses within the day centre sufficient?	Co-researchers/literature
10. Do you feel that you have sufficient knowledge and skills to care for your paediatric patients?	Jenny/literature
11. If you do not have a paediatric background, do you think that you have sufficient support from your peers when caring for children?	Loretta
12. What advantages can you identify regarding the introduction of a specific day for paediatric patients (for the child/the parent/staff/you/ day centre/other units)?	Nina/Loretta
13. What do you see as the disadvantages (for the child/the parent/staff/day centre/other units)?	Nina/Loretta
14. What changes/resources would be needed to support a day dedicated to children?	Co-researchers
15. Is there anything else you would like to add?	Nina

Table 8.4: Development of the patient/parent/child questionnaire.

CLIENT QUESTIONNAIRE DEVELOPMENT	
Question	**Derivative**
1. Who are you?	Co-researchers
2. Should adults/children attend on the same day?	Co-researchers/literature
3. Should there be one day of the week specifically for younger people only?	Co-researchers/literature
4. Why do you think it may be a good idea to have a separate day?	Co-researchers
5. Why do you think it may not be a good idea?	Co-researchers

development, including the demonstration of rigour through objective measures of validity and reliability. Yet she could appreciate the need for a new paradigmatic approach to questionnaire development based on the systematic integration of local, subjective, shared and clinical practice experiences and supportive literature sources. She acknowledged that involvement in an action research project enabled 'us all to learn together' (field note). This confidence, told to me after one of the meetings, was refreshing and supportive of the clinical change process.

The development of the patient/child/carer questionnaire, was (as in the first study) created in-house (table 8.4). This seemed appropriate, as O'Connor (1997, 11) believes 'many tools and approaches have been developed to assist us in helping our clients make difficult decisions. However, the jury is still out regarding their effectiveness, efficiency and suitability with different groups under different circumstances.' Four specific questions were agreed. The most difficult to construct was question number 1. There was much debate regarding how not to offend an adolescent.

> Loretta: *Are we putting 'child'? Not 'child' - young person? Age range? Under 18?*

Many different alternatives were provided, including:

> Nina: *What about 'adults' and 'young people'?* [much laughter]

I explained that in the first study the co-researchers had used the Gobbledegook test (Gunning 1968) to ensure that the patient information that they had produced was pitched at an appropriate reading level. We tried out the test on the patients' questionnaire:

> Patsy: *I scored 19; it's all in nice plain English.*
> Loretta: *Is 19 a bit too low? The* Sun *scores 26! But I suppose how would you feel about your child coming in for surgery? When you've got high anxiety levels, it's very difficult to concentrate, isn't it?*
> Nina: *Let's keep it simple.*

Questionnaire feedback

The staff questionnaire was revised twice (table 8.5 is the final version). Minor changes were made in response to feedback from DSU staff and comments from two paediatric lecturer-practitioners, one based at the Hospital for Sick Children, Great Ormond Street NHS Trust and the other at Guy's and St Thomas' NHS Hospital Trust.

Table 8.5: Staff questionnaire.

COLLABORATIVE ACTION RESEARCH PROJECT

STAFF QUESTIONNAIRE - CARE Of CHILDREN (PAEDIATRIC PROVISION)

Your views are welcomed regarding service provision within the unit. Currently adults and children are admitted to the unit on the same day. Whilst it is acknowledged that staff do specifically consider the differences in care for both groups there is a need to explore whether any improvements to the service a) may be desired and b) are feasible.

To gauge the views of staff and to identify the need for action would you please complete this anonymous questionnaire at your earliest convenience and leave it at the collection point by   . Patients', children's and their carers' views will also be sought.

Please tick your response to each question as required and comment as appropriate.

1.   Please indicate your status (please tick).

                     clerical staff ....
                     consultant anaesthetist ....

(contd)

consultant surgeon ....
health care assistant...............................
nurse ....
ODA ....
porter ....
other ....

2.   Should there be a day dedicated to the needs of paediatric patients?
     (please tick one)

     Yes: No: Don't know:

3.   If you believe that there should be a day dedicated specifically for children
     how often should this occur: (please tick one or comment)

                         once a week
                         fortnightly
                         monthly
                         every six weeks
                         other (please state)

4.   If you are satisfied with the present arrangement please say why.

5.   Which day of the week would appear to be the most suitable to be
     dedicated to children and why?

6.   Which age group do you think is appropriate to attend on this day?
     (please tick one or comment)

                         1–10 years
                         1–13 years
                         1–16 years
                         other - please state:

7.   Should there also be a specific paediatric pre-admission clinic?
     (please tick one)

     Yes: No: Don't know:

8.   If you agree that there should be a paediatric pre-admission clinic, on
     which day of the week should it be held and why?

9.   Is the proportion of paediatric nurses within the day centre sufficient?
     (please tick one)

     Yes: No: Don't know:

10. Do you feel that you have sufficient knowledge and skills to care for your paediatric patients?   (please tick one)

Yes: No: Don't know: Not applicable:

11. If you do not have a paediatric background, do you feel that you have sufficient support from your peers when caring for children? (please tick one)

Yes: No: Don't know: Not applicable:

12. What advantages can you identify regarding the introduction of a specific day for paediatric patients?

For the child:

For the parent/s:

For the staff:

For you:

For the day centre:

For other staff/units:

13. What do you see as the disadvantages of a dedicated day for children?

For the child:

For the parent/s:

For the staff:

For you:

For the day centre:

For other staff/units:

14. What changes/resources would be needed to support a day dedicated to children?

15. Is there anything else that you would like to add?

Thank you for your comments

Loretta: *I did ask you to try out that* [staff] *question-naire, and I don't know if you have had the opportunity.*
Patsy: *I have. I gave it out to the girls.*
Loretta: *Shall we read these out? We need to see how easy the questionnaire was to fill in and whether people would complete it all.*
Rebecca: *The ones I have shown it to were all quite clear. They thought it was all quite simple and easy to follow - they are happy to fill it in as and when we give it to them. And for the patients' questionnaire there was just this bit here: they felt an accompanying parent, guardian, carer would be better.*

The staff and user questionnaires were also sent for comment to the DSU manager, the theatre manager and to the clinical director of the DSU. I received feedback via two telephone calls. I recorded key points within my reflective journal. I considered that the conversations reflected a defensive stance on their part and increasing frustration on mine.

The DSU manager said that, while she could live with the format of the staff questionnaire, she felt the introductory instructions were insufficient. There was a need to convey to current staff that they were doing a good job. She suggested that we should state that the care that is currently provided for children and adults is of a good standard within the constraints of the DSU.

The theatre manager revealed that she had followed the directions of the director of patient services (her manager) and forwarded the staff questionnaire to the Audit Department for comments. She felt that the response could now negate the use of the questionnaire. I acknowledged the usefulness of the information from the Audit Department yet explained why the tool could still be used specifically within the DSU. I believed that there was another reason for suggesting (as I saw it) the termination of the study and challenged her outright. 'What is the problem? Is there potentially so much resistance that we shouldn't proceed?' I was told that she had discovered that the co-researchers' identified problem was, unknown to her, a politically sensitive issue within the Trust. (Neither of us received a satisfactory explanation for this.) She told me that the need to create a dedicated day for children was identified in the strategic plan for the new DSU but had never been put into action. While we both knew that many strategies do not reach fruition, I felt that this disclosure validated the need for further action. However, she continued, 'If this gets out we could lose all our paediatrics to P. hospital.'

The theatre manager also had a message to convey to me from the clinical director of the DSU. She supported the distribution of the staff questionnaire. However, a covering note from senior management to accompany the staff questionnaire was being compiled (box 8.1). This was to reassure staff that the current standard for paediatrics was acceptable and subsequently any changes to current practice were more likely to be considered on a long-term rather than a short-term basis. I was asked to submit the names of all the medical staff who would receive a questionnaire. Also, I was advised not to elicit patients' views at this time.

Box 8.1: Cover note from senior management to accompany the staff questionnaire.

The following questionnaire has been devised by the Day Surgery Unit (DSU) staff following group discussions where they shared their ideas, knowledge and beliefs about how the quality of care for patients could be further enhanced within the DSU. This approach to improving quality of care is strongly supported by the X. Hospitals Trust, and the enthusiasm with which the DSU staff have become involved with the project is to be applauded.

The findings from this questionnaire will be a good grounding on which to base changes and improvements to our service over the next five years as the trust moves forward to a new hospital development. The resultant action plan will therefore be formulated with realistic targets in line with the Trust's overall service context.

This longitudinal approach should in no way devalue the project or the effort put in by the DSU staff. It is hoped that their work will form the basis on which we plan to bring about change and improvements to our already very successful DSU.

What to tell the co-researchers

I took a rather negative view of the telephone calls. Politically, for the managers to be seen to be supporting the project would present the impression of a dynamic organisation which was keen to be innovative, addressing the quality of care and seen to put patients first. Yet, even if the questionnaire responses demonstrated a real need for change, there was no commitment to do so for many years. Strategically, long-termism had been adopted. It was difficult at this stage to decipher whose vested interests were being met to retain the status quo.

I also felt that the new DSU manager had no desire to change. I found her attitude and behaviour very challenging. By non-participation in the project she maintained her distance both from her staff and from me. The only opportunities to discuss her views (apart from the telephone call referred to on page 194) were prior to the co-researcher meetings and feedback to her one hour later. I tried to elicit her interest by emphasising how the group welcomed the opportunity to discuss their views regarding day-surgery nursing and enjoyed shared learning. She was provided with the reading material regarding the quality of paediatric care in a DSU. She articulated why she felt that the standard of child care was adequate within the constraints of the DSU. She stated that everyone was doing their best to provide a good service and that children could be screened from adults. There was no need to currently change the system of organisation. I was forced to confront her resistance to change. I found it difficult to foresee a way forward without her support. Indeed, the need for support from the unit and ward nurse managers had previously been recognised and valued in the first study.

However, while the DSU manager appeared detached and indifferent, both the theatre manager and the clinical director supported the change in principle. Indeed, at the fourth co-researcher meeting the clinical director shared her views:

> CD: *But I think the major constraints are when people have operating lists and when people have outpatients clinics, and it would be very difficult to change those.*
> Loretta: *Yes, I am sure we are all very aware of that, and we do appreciate that with any change process there may well be major problems.*
> CD: *Oh, I don't deny that at all. We have been through a number of changes in the trust, which have been quite painful and nobody would in any way dispute that, but, because we have such a disparate group of surgeons ... the complexities of sorting out surgeons' timetables to try to ensure that children are only brought in on one or one and a half days a week could be difficult.*
> Loretta: *I think it may be that at the end of the day that it is possible; we could say every six weeks this particular day would be a paediatric day ... so it may well be that there is some sort of compromise.*
> CD: *Yes that sort of compromise could possibly be ... I don't have a problem with having a paediatric day ... I am concerned about patients admitted for termination of pregnancy alongside children, it seems that some of*

> *our gynaecological colleagues haven't quite understood why ... The ENT surgeons and certainly one of the ENT anaesthetists are not terribly happy with the current service in the DSU ... the ENT anaesthetist would be a reasonable vehicle to bring about change. I think the surgeons on the whole don't care twopence really as long as they get their caseload through. I think the anaesthetists and the nursing staff are more concerned ... it is the logistics that I am grappling with. I am certainly very keen to have a day's work with paediatric surgery.*

At the next meeting I shared the nature of the telephone calls as well as my current reservations. The co-researchers' response was a truly enlightening experience for me. Their perception was the antithesis of mine. First, they were absolutely delighted that 'their little project' was having such a resounding impact at all levels of the organisation.

> Rebecca: *It's brilliant that we have ruffled so many feathers, especially up there.*
> Jenny: *It's great and truly amazing that little we, the workers, who are never consulted about anything, should have caused such a stir! They've had to sit up and take notice.* [much laughter]
> Nina: *It shows you how small steps can have major effects.*

The effect on the co-researchers

The co-researchers saw themselves as powerless subordinates, but their reaction demonstrated the experience of power. This could equate with what Torbert (1991) refers to as 'liberating structures', which cultivate empowerment through development. The cover note (box 8.1), which would accompany the staff questionnaire, was perceived by the co-researchers as supportive of their efforts to date. They were content to accept a long-term view. Although:

> Chris: *Will we be around in five years' time?*

A less positive response was seen to the DSU manager's comments regarding the current 'good' service for all patients. The co-researchers were reluctant to agree to this. We eventually agreed to write on the introductory section of the staff questionnaire:

> While it is acknowledged that staff do specifically consider the differences in care for both groups (adults and children), there is a need to explore whether any improvements to the service may (a) be desired and (b) be feasible.

I explored the theatre manager's feedback with the co-researchers. Nina and I agreed that the Audit Department's comments regarding the staff questionnaire were predictable. I broached the politically sensitive issue:

> Loretta: *I said: 'Now tell me, K. [TM], just tell me what is all this about?' She said if it gets out that the DSU here doesn't have a specific day for children, and another one does, for example at P. hospital, then there is competition. GPs might decide to refer children there, or parents may say: 'Oh, they specifically cater for children at P. hospital; they don't here. You know how these things get out and people start talking.' It's interesting, isn't it? Because you try and anticipate, as we have been doing, possible reasons for resistance to change, but I must admit I didn't anticipate that at all! Mind you, I would have thought it was a key reason to change!*
> Patsy: *I think a lot of the parents that come here do know that there is a children's unit at P. hospital, but they are happy with the care here.*
> Rebecca: *A* [the clinical director] *wants to support a paediatric day and obviously wants to promote this new unit.*

It was with much regret that we put the patients' questionnaire on hold. We tried to reconcile ourselves to management's dilemma. On the one hand, the Trust may have wished to advocate patient partnership and participation in care yet, on the other hand, we were deterred from exploring potential inadequacies of current service provision for fear of losing patients to a neighbouring Trust. Ovretveit (1997) recognises that involving (or in our case attempting to involve) patients in decision-making can, like sharing information, bring professions (and others) into closer co-operation or conflict.

Moving forward

The motivation to continue with the study was enhanced by openly sharing our perceptions of the change process. Also, it appeared that the co-researchers were even more committed and determined to advance the initiative in spite of, or as a result of, management's reticence.

> Rebecca: *The more we are getting into this and the more resentment we are getting from the hierarchy, the more I believe we should continue.*
> Nina: *They need to know how strongly we feel about this issue.*

There was much discussion regarding implementation of the staff questionnaire, which had to be delayed because of the prolonged consultation process. We decided to send the questionnaires to all the staff who were currently employed to work in the DSU, except for the bank nurses. The bank nurses worked irregular and fewer hours and replaced staff on an infrequent basis. The sample consisted of 86 members of staff (see table 8.6).

Table 8.6: DSU staff who received a questionnaire.

Member of Staff (alphabetical order)	Number currently employed
Anaesthetists	11
Clerical staff	6
Healthcare assistants	4
Nurses	34
Operating department personnel	6
Porter	1
Surgeons	24

Distribution of the staff questionnaire was eventually to occur in January (while I was on leave). As in the first study excited anticipation tinged with anxiety was evident:

> Jenny: *On the sixteenth, we are on a roll.*
> Rebecca: *If a surgeon comes into the building, we will be in the cupboard!* [laughter]

I shared my reflections of the first action research study regarding potential resistors to change, especially the anaesthetists (see page 119). The advice from Raelin (1989) regarding achieving co-operation from physicians (page 153) was especially appropriate. I offered to compile a second accompaniment to the staff questionnaire (the first being the letter from senior management, box 8.1) entitled: 'What's in it for us?' which explained the action research process of gaining co-operation and collaboration. It was difficult for us, at this stage, to clearly identify the specific benefits to staff. Question number 12 (table 8.5) enables staff to identify the advantages of the proposed change for the patients, for themselves and for the DSU. We hoped that this approach would reinforce the need for congruent professional and organisational values regarding the necessity for change.

> Loretta: *Basically, most people don't want to change. It's much easier just to hang on and so you have to try to make an overwhelming case for change, and they have to believe in it and want to do it.*

Chapter 9

Descriptive analysis of the unfreezing process

'Whatever you decide to do, you must be open about it
with the whole workforce.' (Smith 1996)

This chapter continues to explore the perspectives of the day surgery
unit (DSU) staff regarding the proposed innovation, the creation of a
dedicated day for children's surgery. An analysis of the data from the
staff questionnaire is provided as well as an interpretation of the
findings. This descriptive analysis also encompasses the co-researchers'
perceptions, personal reflections and insights from the DSU staff who
attended a questionnaire-feedback meeting. Present at the feedback
meeting were the theatre manager, 15 nurses, two operating department personnel, myself and three of the co-researchers.

Approaches to data analysis

The use of a questionnaire in an action research study is, according to
Stringer (1996), a valid approach to inquiry. However, the analysed
data should be used purely for description.

> The meaning or significance of any of the information
> can only be determined by the people who live the
> culture of the setting, who have the profound under-
> standing that comes from extended immersion in the
> ongoing social and cultural life of that context ... We
> come closer to the reality of other people's experience
> and, in the process, increase the potential for creating
> truly effective services and programs that will enhance
> the lives of the people we serve. (Stringer 1996, 157-
> 158)

Insiders and outsiders may analyse the data together (Bartunek and Louis 1996). One party may provide a tentative interpretation, and the other may critique and advance the interpretation. Three of the co-researchers met to start to analyse the data (while I was on leave), which they presented at the next co-researcher meeting.

> Loretta: *So you managed to analyse them* [the questionnaires] *as well?*
> Nina: *Well, Rebecca and I met, and then Patsy helped me with a bit. It is not an in-depth analysis - just counting up the numbers and then trying to collate them.*

Response rate

All the questionnaires that were returned were analysed. However, not all the respondents answered every question.

No. of questionnaires sent:	86
No. of questionnaires returned:	50
Response rate:	58%

The response rate reflects Robinson's (1989) assertion that a 50%-60% response rate is the best to be expected if no follow-up letter is issued. However, the co-researchers were at hand to remind their peers to complete their form. They were not disappointed with the outcome. They were especially pleased with the response rate from the nurses, see table 9.1, which at 73% was 'very good' (Robinson 1989).

Of all the responses, we had hoped for a higher return rate of questionnaires from the surgeons and anaesthetists. However, the theatre manager was impressed with the overall outcome, especially from the 18

Table 9.1: Sample response rate.

Sample	No. sent	No. returned	Response rate
Anaesthetists	11	6	54%
Clerical staff	6	3	50%
Healthcare assistants	4	2	50%
Nurses	34	25	73%
Operating department personnel	6	1	16%
Porter	1	1	100%
Surgeons	24	12	50%

medical staff, who had, she declared, *'Taken the trouble to reply'* (field note). Her past experience of surveys in healthcare settings was that there was usually a very low response rate. This view had recently been reinforced to her by personnel within the Audit Department.

Until I saw the sample response rate I had not appreciated that Chris (co-researcher) had been unsupported by her peers in the operating department (non-nurses). No other member of the operating department personnel had responded to the questionnaire. She became rather defensive:

> Chris: *I really don't think it mattered that much to them. However, the porter told me that he was delighted to be given the opportunity to share his views.*

A specific day for children

Question number 2 (see table 8.5, p. 192) regarding whether there should be a day dedicated to children demonstrated that overall slightly more respondents felt the need for a dedicated day; more nurses supported this view (see table 9.2 below).

> Nina: *I was quite pleasantly surprised that it balanced out, because there were as many people for it as against it.*

It appeared that the majority of medical staff respondents wished to retain the status quo.

Table 9.2: DSU staff responses to whether there should there be a day dedicated to the needs of children.

Question: Do you think there should be a day dedicated to children?

	23 (46%) **Yes**	21 (42%) **No**	6 (12%) **Don't know**
Nurse	14	8	3
Surgeon	3	7	2
Anaesthetist	3	2	1
Healthcare assistant	1	1	–
Operating department assistant	1	-	–
Clerical	–	3	–
Porter	1	–	–

> Patsy: *Well, the total response of the medical staff was satisfactory, but only six of these think that it is a good idea.*

However, I felt that six was a good start, and, also, there were another three who were unsure. I thought it possible that the more motivated staff could create the opportunity to pilot the innovation.

Fifty percent of the respondents agreed to a specified day to be held once a month. Interestingly, although two members of staff (one nurse and one surgeon) felt negative about a paediatric day, they both responded to this question. One day a month had previously been identified in the literature (see table 8.2, page 184). When asked which would be the preferred day (of the month), there were mixed views. The most popular day was Friday. Saturday was the next most popular choice although, at that time, the DSU only operated Monday-Friday! However, this day was a logical choice as the possibility of extending the working week to enable effective use of resources had been aired with the DSU staff. Respondents could also identify the potential benefits of a Saturday for school children and working carers.

There was no problem identifying the lower age range for children. The DSU accepted children from the age of one year. However, what should be the upper age limit? When does an older child become a young adult? The majority of respondents (see table 9.3) shared the view of an anaesthetist:

> *Appropriate age range to be treated for children 1-13 without feeling they are embarrassed. Over 13 can be integrated with adults.*

Table 9.3: Respondents' views on the appropriate age range for paediatric day attendance.

Age	Surgeons	Anaesthetists	Nurses	Total
1–10	3	2	2	7
1–13	–	2	13	15
1–16	1	–	4	5

It was important to assess the perspectives of staff regarding the current arrangement in the DSU (question number 4, table 8.5, p. 192). It was apparent that maintaining the status quo for the medical staff was the least disruptive option for them. The medical staff felt that children's needs were met most of the time. They felt that the current system was effective for the booking of patients. However, subsequent comments suggested that a revision of workloads should be undertaken, i.e there were insufficient children for each surgeon to have a complete list; consequently, the DSU was not being fully utilised. One surgeon suggested that a specific children's day and the resultant organisational change would 'further alienate staff'.

Opposing views

From the nurses' data there are clearly two opposing views. The current arrangements appeared to work well, and if there was a specific day more resources were seen to be required, e.g. increased staff, more theatre equipment and a bigger play room. One respondent felt the ability to change was impossible - *'consultants would be hard to pin down and the place would be overrun with children'*. Another respondent stated that with a few children in at a time there is always a paediatric nurse giving practically 1–1 care. Another nurse felt that safety could be maintained (because of the small throughput of children). These assertions are the antithesis of the co-researchers' reflections on practice. Jenny's perceptions of care and Chris's personal experience of the preparation of inappropriate theatre instruments (see pages 177–178) refute the view that all is well.

Opposing views clearly demonstrated the need for improvement. Current guidelines on child care in DSUs needed to be identified, and there was recognition that general trained nurses were not happy caring for paediatrics. There was also a recognised need to explore the views of patients. These initial comments were elaborated upon in questions 12 and 13, table 8.5, p. 193), which requested that respondents identify the advantages and disadvantages of a dedicated day for children, parents, the DSU staff, each member of the DSU, the DSU and other staff/units.

The advantages/disadvantages of a specified day for children

The advantageous themes for the child reflected a child-friendly unit, enhanced management and provision of holistic care. Respondents felt that being with other children would result in a more friendly, less formal environment where children could mix more freely. To further reduce anxiety/psychological stress, balloons, music, decorations and no uniforms were felt to create the appropriate environment. There would be an appropriate concentration of resources specifically for children, with better organisation of operating lists. The need for surgery and anaesthetics to be performed by consultants and anaesthetists with special skills/knowledge of paediatrics reflected previous findings in the literature (see page 183).

My son has been to P. hospital's Day Treatment Centre, and, although care was lousy, the atmosphere was much more relaxed and geared towards the care of children, e.g. balloons etc. As a parent I would be very upset to see adults being cared for in the same area. We should be able to provide a more child-friendly environment.

The perceived disadvantages of a specific day for children reflected these two themes: reduced standard of care and physical restrictions. It was felt that if there were more children in the DSU they would each receive less attention from paediatric nurses. This may increase their anxiety and stress as they may not be appropriately cared for. The co-researchers felt that this was a weak argument considering paediatric nurses are currently not always on duty when children are present. Other perceived disadvantages included increased upset due to witnessing other children in distress, and inadequate pain control during and after discharge. Both these issues could currently occur. At the feedback meeting to DSU staff it was felt that these events were less likely to happen with all staff focused on children's needs.

The physical restrictions were considered valid. These included a concern that with a set day once a month there was no flexibility/ opportunity to change. Yet this could also be viewed as forward planning. With a specific future date the home situation could be appropriately organised. Also, the waiting list could potentially be lengthened. One surgeon questioned how to prioritise who is first/last on the operating list. Another identified disadvantages related to the small play area. Rebecca highlighted for her peers (at the DSU feedback meeting) a previous discussion by the co-researchers regarding the possibility of almost all the DSU becoming a potential play area (as had occurred at the previous, but now closed, DSU). This idea was viewed with initial alarm and then considered interest.

For the parents/carers, there were also diverse views regarding psychological support versus inadequate support, and physical care versus physical restrictions. The respondents felt that with a specified day parents were more able to meet and support one another. They could exchange ideas, fears and knowledge. It should be reassuring for them to see a unit altered to specifically care for their children. Yet other respondents felt that there would be a lack of support for parents related to a lack of understanding by staff. There may be less individual care for the child and no time for effective communication. Once again physical restrictions referred to the potential for overcrowding, as well as raised noise levels. Yet other staff felt that it would be easier for parents to look after their children. Currently, when parents accompany their child to the anaesthetic and recovery areas they are often aware of intruding on adult patients' privacy.

What were the potential advantages and disadvantages for the DSU staff? The most significant outcome from the data reflected attitudes to children. It was clear that some staff do not like looking after children. Children were viewed as being very noisy, taking longer to admit, assess and reassure, and as creating 'chaos'. Yet the more positive respondents recognised that, even if you were not keen on children, *'it's over in a day!'* Also, off duty could be altered accordingly. It would clearly be a focused day in which all staff could concentrate solely on the child. With no adults to care for, more time could be devoted to children. There would be more appropriate use of the three paediatric nurses and a 'play leader' could possibly be employed (or shared with the children's ward). There would be consideration for TOP (termination of pregnancy) patients who may currently be nursed alongside children. Crying from children would not distress adult patients, which was a common occurrence. Staff communication should be enhanced.

Besides negative attitudes to children (see above), negative perspectives reflected the changes in working practice. These included *'a heavy day'*, the perceived difficulty in reorganising the unit and the need for surgeons agreeing to who would operate on their patients. Resource implications included a lack of adequate equipment, the need for adequate staff training to ensure competence and confidence and a perceived lack of staff. These views were explored at the feedback meeting. There was recognition of some misconceptions regarding attitudes to children. However, the TM felt that there could be some flexibility regarding which nurses were on duty, especially as this could potentially be planned on a monthly basis. She also reassured the staff that they would receive further education and training regarding the care of children.

It was also equally important to gauge how each member of the DSU staff personally viewed the potential change. There were similar positive responses which reflected a safe environment, personal enlightenment and education. Respondents perceived that there would always be support from paediatric nurses and the facilities would be child-focused. The opportunity to devote more time to children's needs was considered, including becoming more experienced at assessing their pain levels. Overall, more experience with children would increase knowledge, skills and confidence in paediatric nursing; subsequently, stress levels should be reduced. Yet the disadvantages far outweighed the advantages, especially from the medical staff's perspective. Surgeons stated that a dedicated day may not fit in with other commitments, may make planning difficult, would be boring and they may only have a half-filled list (they topped up with adult patients). There would be increased responsibility, it would be tiring and it would take extra time to prepare the unit and become familiar with families. All these perceived disadvantages appear to position the healthcare professional's needs before those of the patient/user/consumer. Only six members of staff stated that there would be no disadvantages to themselves.

The perceived advantages and disadvantages of a specified day for the DSU, and for other staff/clinical areas within the Trust, reflect many of the previous comments. Additional views included a more efficient approach to managing the unit and marketing the service. Yet the overall value of a change in practice was succinctly identified by an anaesthetist:

> *Our only motivation should be improving things for the child.*

Paediatric pre-admission clinic

The inclusion of questions regarding a pre-admission clinic specifically for children (table 8.5, p. 192) reflects Rebecca's astute observation (see page 175) and the number one standard within the CCHS (1991) guidelines (see table 8.1, page 183). At the feedback meeting Rebecca also explained the importance of both a specified day and a pre-admission clinic:

> *When a dedicated day list ran at X. hospital, it worked very well. The ward was decorated with balloons etc., the staff wore civilian clothes ... the nurses who pre-assessed the children on a Saturday morning at X. were on duty for the day of operation. This helped greatly with forming a relationship with child and parents.*

Twenty-nine members of staff agreed with the development of a paediatric pre-admission clinic. Of the nine respondents who disagreed, two felt that this was a more feasible option than a specified day. One of the four nurses who was not sure requested more guidance in the way of information leaflets, books, videos, etc. for parents to better prepare their children pre-admission.

Jenny reflected on the reassuring outcome of the feedback meeting:

> *They all thought it was a good idea to have a special pre-admission clinic.*

For the nurses the most popular day for the clinic was Saturday, the same as the specified day for surgery, and for similar reasons regarding school and carers working. The staff at the feedback meeting felt that a Saturday was likely to be a more relaxing experience for children and carers. There would be no other patients in the DSU and potentially both carers and any number of siblings could accompany them. However, there was some concern regarding the availability of a surgeon and an anaesthetist on a Saturday, to be on hand to discuss any significant problems identified by the nurses. Indeed, this could be a potential problem. The days identified by the medical staff varied and reflected their current availability. One anaesthetist felt that she did not know which day would best suit all concerned but was convinced that a pre-admission clinic would be *'less intimidating for the children than with lots of strange adults around'*.

Paediatric support

Respondents were asked to identify their current perceptions of 'support' in caring for children in the day surgery setting. Support referred to paediatric nurses employed in the unit (question number 9), the respondents' knowledge and skills of paediatric care (question number 10) and peer support (question 11). Very few of the sample (7) believed that the proportion of paediatric nurses in the DSU was sufficient.

The nurses in particular felt that there was a lack of trained paediatric nurses. Recruiting paediatric nurses is a national problem. Consequently, to ensure a good quality of service provision for children, general nurses need to be provided with specific paediatric knowledge and skills. Indeed, many of the respondents (14) in question ten, identified gaps in knowledge (see table 9.4 below).

Table 9.4: Perceptions of sufficient knowledge and skills to care for paediatric patients.

Question: Do you think you possess sufficient knowledge and skills for paediatric care?

	Yes	No	Don't know	Not applicable
Porter	1	–	–	–
Operating department assistant	1	–	–	–
Healthcare assistant	–	2	–	–
Anaesthetist	5	1	–	–
Surgeon	7	1	–	2
Nurse	10	10	1	2

Of the medical staff, one anaesthetist admitted that she felt confident caring for children but not babies. A surgeon wrote that he only did procedures that he considered simple, 'the rest go to P. hospital'.

While a gap in knowledge was identified by 14 staff, during discussion at the feedback meeting this number significantly increased. The TM, as a priority, agreed to review education provision for DSU staff.

The extent to which there was peer support was also explored (question 11). Table 9.5 reflects the response. The most significant response is to be found in the surgeon column. Of the ten surgeons who responded to this question, five felt they did receive sufficient peer support, while five felt that the question did not apply to them! For the nurses, only ten felt sufficiently supported by their peers.

Table 9.5: Respondents' view of sufficient peer support.

Question: Do you believe you receive sufficient peer support?

	Yes	No	Don't know	Not applicable
Porter	1	–	–	–
Operating department assistant	1	–	–	–
Healthcare assistant	1	–	1	1
Anaesthetist	4	1	–	–
Surgeon	5	–	–	5
Nurse	10	4	1	3

Perceived changes required for a dedicated paediatric day

Having explored views on the key issues of moving to a specific day for children (and a pre-admission clinic), the respondents were asked, in question 14 (table 8.5, p. 193) to summarise the specific changes required. The perceived changes encompassed four broad areas:

- appropriate staff
- physical environment
- new ways of working
- attitude change

Overall, there was a need for more paediatric nurses, surgeons and anaesthetists. Innovative comments included utilising the skills of a play leader and/or nursery nurse and a consideration of a 24-hour after-care service via a paediatric community link nurse. Further education for current staff was a recurring theme.

Many comments referred to strategies for altering and enhancing the physical environment. A risk assessment of the unit for children was advocated. The decor should be more child-friendly with a bigger play area. Nurses should wear tabards and remove their theatre caps in the recovery area. More emergency equipment and operating instruments may be required. Innovative ideas included the provision of a separate medicine cupboard for drugs containing paediatric dosages. Also, a system of awards for children could be provided on discharge, e.g. presentation of a DSU certificate and/or cartoon plasters etc.

The leadership and management of new ways of working was advocated for all DSU staff. There was clear support for a pre-admission clinic. Admissions should be controlled by the DSU in co-operation with consultants. Surgeons would need to agree who would operate on a specific day. Saturday was once again identified as the most appropriate day, as it was felt that there would be less disruption for patients, carers and staff. Children should be given set appointment times, with younger children given priority on the operating list. There was also support for an ongoing audit of paediatric service provision.

Some respondents felt that the basic resources required would not incur large costs. Small costs were a positive feature of adaptation identified by Nicholl et al. (1996). It was felt that an enthusiastic attitude would be a positive motivator for change. Indeed, attitudes were clearly in evidence in the final question (number 15), which gave respondents the opportunity to include anything else they wished to say. Once again both positive and negative responses could be identified.

The nurses' comments ranged from 'no go' to the pleasure at being asked for their opinion. A member of staff who recalled working with dedicated paediatric day surgery lists declared that the benefits to parents, child and staff: 'FAR OUTWEIGH ANY DISADVAN-TAGES' (respondent's capitals).

A final negative comment from a member of the medical staff needs to be considered alongside a positive perspective:

> Surgeon: *I have answered the only useful question which is number 2. The rest is paediatric ideology.*
> Anaesthetist: *When can we start? I applaud this initiative - good luck.*

Chris's final comment seemed to capture a belief that appeared to be shared by some of the questionnaire respondents and was supported by the staff at the feedback meeting:

> Chris: *This can work if properly and carefully planned, with full consultation between staff, management, anaesthetists and surgeons.*

Co-researchers' reflections

I discussed with the co-researchers their overall views of the questionnaire and the need for a further action plan.

> Nina: *I think some of the reasons why those that were against it seemed to be against it are fairly legitimate, but it doesn't mean to say that maybe there isn't enough people for it that you could actually start in some slow way organising a clinic with those people that were interested and then that may snowball. People see it as just an obstruction at the moment, don't they? Too many things to change to do it.*
>
> Chris: *I think also that if somebody has had no experience of a day dedicated to paediatric surgery, it was difficult for them to make an objective comment about it. The ones that seem to be positive are the ones that have experienced it before at X. hospital. There are some really good points that have come out of it. Could we write a report or something?*
>
> Loretta: *Yes, there will be a report, but I was just wondering: an interim measure for the staff?*
>
> Rebecca: *Can we feed back the results to the staff? It would be nice for them to see.*
>
> Loretta: *I couldn't agree more. I think that would be very worthwhile and interesting to hear what people have to say.*
>
> Nina: *We have got almost half for and half against, and all the against are related to the logistics of changing it. We could say that there seems to be quite strong support for it and therefore feel it's worthwhile exploring the views of patients, parents and children - see what they think.*

I wished to feed back the questionnaire results to the DSU staff at the earliest opportunity. Fortunately, the DSU manager was able to provide me with a 'slot' at the next staff meeting. However, she remarked that she would not be able to stay for the feedback presentation.

Feeding back the findings

The theatre manager was present at the feedback meeting to the staff of the DSU. Although the DSU manager was on duty, she conveyed apologies for her absence. Fifteen nurses and two operating department personnel were present as well as co-researchers Rebecca, Jenny and Chris. I took the decision not to audiotape the meeting. I felt the staff might view the micro-cassette with suspicion especially with a senior manager present. In retrospect I wished I had asked permission to tape the meeting as the presentation of the data analysis generated worthwhile discussions and creative insights. There was also much amusement as staff recognised their specific comments. As well as feeding back the results from the questionnaires the meeting also enabled the co-researchers and me to provide detailed information regarding national guidelines and recent developments regarding the care of children in DSUs.

> DSU nurse: *If only we'd known that we wouldn't have been so negative.* (field note)

Discussions centred around the costs and benefits of an enhanced paediatric service. Nurses acknowledged that they needed to appreciate the whole situation - not just other colleagues' views but also those of parents and children. There was much interest in advancing knowledge regarding paediatric care. The DSU staff also explored the changes that might be required to convert to a dedicated day; many creative ideas continued to emerge. The consensus was that changes to the physical environment were manageable. I started to feel reassured by their increasingly positive responses.

> DSU nurse: *Is this it? What will happen next? Nothing?* (field note)

I asked the staff to identify a way forward, and they quickly responded with four proposals:

- investigate the views of children and parents/carers about the current service, include their views on both proposed initiatives (dedicated day and pre-admission clinic)

- explore the educational needs of each member of staff regarding the care of children
- pilot a dedicated day or half-day with surgeons and anaesthetists who are supportive of the initiative
- create a specific paediatric pre-admission clinic

By the end of the meeting it was apparent that the discussion reinforced the need for change for the already committed members of staff. Lancaster and Lancaster (1982) refer to active accepters or rejectors, passive accepters or rejectors and noncommitted individuals. The staff who had not been initially enthusiastic felt that they now had much more insight into the nature of the project and could appreciate the need for change.

The TM could not stay for the whole discussion and left towards the end of the meeting. Yet she noted the comments regarding the need for further education and informed the staff that I would be writing an interim report for further management consideration. She very much valued the meeting.

> TM to the DSU staff: *We've been able to talk about nursing, we never really have time to discuss those crucial issues. This is a real eye opener for me!* (field note)

As I left the meeting I noted one final supportive comment:

> DSU staff nurse to me: *We'll invite you to the first day dedicated to children!* (field note)

The possibility for change

It seemed a natural end to the study as it appeared that I would not be able to take the initiative any further forward (owing to senior management's long-term view). I felt disappointed that I had, in some way, let down the co-researchers. However, the TM offered to explore a collaborative way forward with the clinical director of the DSU:

> *Well, I will certainly sit down with A. and talk through the findings from the questionnaire and the outcome of the feedback session. Even though they* [the co-researchers] *have realistic expectations and they know*

> *that we aren't probably going to get a single paediatric*
> *day next year, we can still make some improvements.*

And what of the vending machine?

As we could not advance the paediatric cause any further, I could only hope that the vending machine issue had been resolved.

> Patsy: *Well, to be honest, I haven't said any more to B.*
> *about it because she has only just settled into the unit;*
> *so I didn't want to bombard her ... I wanted to discuss*
> *what happened when I phoned Coca Cola here first*
> *before going to see her.*
> Loretta: *Well, let's hold onto this until you feel the time*
> *is right to mention it to B. ... I invited her to the meeting*
> *when I spoke to her, but it is probably too soon yet.*

In fact although Patsy had undertaken all the exploratory work the vending machine had still not been installed by the time I withdrew from the study. She had told the DSU manager that the Coca Cola installation charge was to be waived, and that the co-researchers had identified a relevant site for the machine and the safe disposal of recycled cans. Yet:

> Patsy: *I don't think B. is too much against it.* **She's** *still*
> *trying to find a place to put it!*

Moving forward

Analysing and interpreting the questionnaires both independently and with the co-researchers was a rewarding experience for me. Their interpretations enhanced my understanding of the data. Overall, they were content with the response rate and could accommodate most of the negative comments from their peers and medical colleagues. Following clarification and further exploration of the need for change at the DSU feedback meeting, many more of the staff appeared motivated to change. There was evidence of progress from the unfreezing stage towards the next phase of the change process, the 'moving stage' (Lewin 1952). In this phase cognitive redefinition occurs due to collecting sufficient information about the situation and recognising the need to alter the status quo and agreeing an action plan. This was the outcome of the feedback meeting. It was hoped that the suggestions proposed by the staff would be considered. A realistic proposal was initially to work with staff who were motivated to change. The innovations, i.e. a dedicated day and a pre-admission clinic, could then be piloted and evaluated. The theatre manager appeared committed to these future developments for the DSU staff, although the first priority was for education provision.

Chapter 10

A framework to advance change and development in clinical practice

'The main purpose of action research is to bring about an improvement in practice.' (McNiff, Lomax and Whitehead 1996)

Similarities between the first and the second studies are evident. The significance of these similarities became increasingly evident from both the analysis of the process and outcomes of the second study and from further comparison with the first study. Compatible themes emerged that reflected the change experience for the co-researchers in both studies. This was in spite of the fact that the second study had not progressed beyond the unfreezing stage. However, an action research cycle (see table 7.1, p. 168) had been completed in the second study. Also, owing to the delays of the second study, only process outcomes for the co-researchers and the theatre manager could be elicited at this time. Nevertheless, the positive outcomes that emerged from both studies reinforced the need to continue to explore the use of the critical action research approach for nurses in clinical practice. From the analysis, and comparison of the process and outcomes of both studies, a conceptual framework to advance nurse-led change and development in clinical practice was developed.

The analytic process

Fleming and Moloney (1996) compare the differences between analysing interpretive and socially critical data. They suggest that interpretive data, from interview transcripts etc., is collapsed into codes

217

and core categories while the socially critical theorist adopts a different approach by overtly looking for patterns of a socio-political nature (see table 2.6, p. 38). However, in this study, a combined approach to analysis was adopted to enable an enhanced understanding of the nature of the change process from a personal, interpersonal, multi-professional and organisational perspective. Theoretical knowledge informed the analysis of the second study in the day surgery unit (DSU). May (1998) refers to the importance of theory as a lens through which data is interpreted. As in the first study, knowledge from critical social theory, change theory, adult and experiential learning theories, theories of reflection and the collaboration and oppression nursing literature enhanced the analysis of the change process apparent in the second study.

The resultant thematic analysis encompassed data from the co-researcher meetings, the DSU feedback meeting and from field notes and reflective journal entries. The data was repeatedly and systematically examined, coded and clustered. From the analysis 223 codes emerged that were condensed to 42 clusters. The process of coding and clustering reflected the approach that I adopted in the first study (see page 130). Once I had collapsed the codes to clusters of data, I chose to staple each of the 42 clusters (and their associated codes) onto sheets of A3 paper. This flexible approach enabled me, at any free moment, to gain access to all of the data and continue to reflect on my analysis. It also enabled me to collate the 42 clusters into a manageable format for the themes to emerge.

From repeated immersion in the data five key themes eventually emerged, which appeared to represent the critical action research process within the DSU. The five themes that were derived from the clusters were: staff empowerment, disempowerment recognition, demonstrable interpersonal support, personal enhancement and participative facilitation (see table 10.1).

In the first study Lewin's Force Field Analysis categories were used to provide a collective organising framework in which to determine the motivating and modifying change factors (tables 2.1 and 6.1). The same process was used in the second study (table 10.2). The most fundamental construct for Lewin is the 'field'. All behaviour, including action, thinking, wishing, striving, valuing, achieving, etc., is conceived of as a change of some state of a field in a given unit of time (Cartwright 1963).

Table 10.1: Thematic analysis of the derived DSU data.

THE CRITICAL ACTION RESEARCH PROCESS WITHIN THE DSU
(42 clusters, 5 themes)

Staff empowerment
Open communication
Problem identification
Initiating and undertaking action
Multi-professional engagement
Collaborative practice
Doctors' positive feedback
Peers' positive feedback
Evidence from the literature
Management support
Equitable co-researcher participation
Challenging the status quo
Management reticence

Personal Enhancement
Sharing knowledge and beliefs
Learning research
Challenging assumptions
Influencing multi-professional
    assumptions
Seeking information
Collaborative problem-solving
Analysing feedback
Recognising personal growth
Identifying positive outcomes

Disempowerment recognition
Power conflicts
Reading avoidance
Peers' change fatigue
Anonymity constraints
Knowledge deficit
Variable time constraints
Feedback avoidance
Passive acceptance

Demonstrable Interpersonal
    Support
Humour
Digression
Group reflective analysis
Social celebration

Participative Facilitation
Open communication
Risk-taking
Psychological safety
Consideration of the context
Patient focused
Enabling consensus and collaboration
Empathy
Positive reinforcement
Fostering realistic expectations

Undertaking the field analysis provided another perspective in the complexities of change in the second study. It enabled a clear overview of the significant factors that influenced the process of change. When compared with the field analysis from the first study (table 6.1, p. 131), many similarities regarding undertaking change within clinical settings can be elicited.

Table 10.2: The motivating and modifying change factors within the DSU (second study).

Field analysis	Motivating factors	Modifying factors
Technical	Patient focused	Non-user/patient involvement
Economic	'Protected' time	Old ways of working
Political	Medical staff perceptions Challenging the status quo	Power conflicts 'Sensitive issue'
Socio-cultural	Peers' positive feedback Humorous coping Social celebration	Anonymity constraints Digression Change fatigue
Organisational	Management support Management reticence	Oppressive culture Risk analysis
Policy	NHS Trust policy for DSU Literature evidence	Long-termism
Structural	Bottom-up innovation Collaborative meetings	Threat to management Unilateral decisions
Group	Open communication Equitable participation Consensus	Realistic expectations
Interpersonal	Shared beliefs Shared knowledge Reflective action	Psychological safety
Individual/person	Personal-growth recognition 'Pioneers'	Reading avoidance Passive acceptance

Data compatibility

Much of the data within the second study is compatible with that of the first study. Indeed, many of the findings are either identical or very similar, as identified in table 10.3. This is in spite of the fact that the second study ended prematurely. Boyatzis (1998) refers to consistency of judgement in data analysis. He identifies the need for consistency over time and events which is attained when a person makes the same observation at two different times or in two different settings.

Table 10.3: Similarity of data analysis findings within both studies.

First study	Second study
shared reflections	group reflective analysis
collaboration	collaborative practice
power conflicts	power conflicts
knowledge deficit	knowledge deficit
initiating action	initiating and undertaking action
humorous coping	humour
risk-taking	risk-taking
positive anticipation	fostering realistic expectations
positive reinforcement	positive reinforcement
problem-solving	collaborative problem-solving
sharing knowledge	sharing knowledge and beliefs
positive outcomes	identifying positive outcomes
doctors' perceptions	doctors' positive feedback
personal growth	recognising personal growth
psychological safety	psychological safety
digression	digression
time constraints	variable time constraints
feedback avoidance	feedback avoidance

It is interesting to note that in the first study I had reduced clusters of data to categories; in this study I reduced the clusters to themes. There is no difference between the two terms, they are interchangeable (May 1998). However, the term 'thematic analysis' is currently more prevalent within the research literature (Wolcott 1994, Coffey and Atkinson 1996). According to Boyatzis (1998), thematic analysis is an appropriate method for exploring complex, multidisciplinary phenomena. He notes that tolerance of ambiguity is a desired characteristic of the researcher using thematic analysis. Consequently, being an action researcher is congruent with the chosen qualitative data analysis strategy. Learning to live with ambiguity has been a recurrent feature of the two studies.

The first study resulted in 167 codes, 55 clusters and 23 categories. Within the second study there were 223 codes, 42 clusters and 5 themes. The figures demonstrate a developmental process as my confidence in data analysis increased over time. Although the raw data for analysis was far less than in the first study, more codes were elicited. On reflection I can appreciate that the 23 categories from the first study were rather unwieldy. They could certainly have been further reduced. The five themes that have emerged from the second study (see table 10.1, p. 219) encompass findings within both studies (table 10.3). Many of the findings encompass power issues within clinical settings.

Yet it is just these power issues, at many levels of the organisation, which are the most difficult to resolve.

Power issues

By challenging the status quo regarding paediatric day-care provision in the DSU the co-researchers risked conflict at all levels of the organisation. Aspland et al. (1996) suggest that, rather than trying to avoid such problems arising, it is better that one should simply be prepared for such complexities to be considered as integral elements of collaborative research, and to deal with such matter as challenges rather than problems. This appeared to be the case in the second study, in spite of disempowering factors. In the study there are both empowering and disempowering factors associated with nurses, medical staff and managers. These factors encompass the evidence from the literature regarding the perception of nurses as an oppressed group, often portrayed as subservient to medicine, and invisible to management. Yet as significant in the second study was the culture of the NHS Trust, which often resulted in the disempowerment of healthcare staff at differing levels of the organisation. Bertinasco (1990) believes that interpersonal conflicts in hospitals seem to be increasing. He also confirms the extent to which nursing is devalued and disempowered:

> Compared with student nurses who have a relatively
> high image of nurses on average, the general-duty
> nurse has an especially low image of nurses, and other
> hospital personnel have an even lower image of nursing.
> (Bertinasco 1990, 37)

Issues of power and oppression were in evidence on my first encounter with both the theatre manager and the co-researchers.

> TM, new in post: *Basically I was given no choice in the
> matter. I am actually in great favour of collaborative
> work ... but, nonetheless, I didn't have a choice.*

Interestingly, although she felt aggrieved and powerless, she did not ensure that the DSU staff were given freedom of choice; she selected the participants for the study. Nina, the nurse lecturer, chose to partici-pate in the study whereas there was a passive acceptance to comply by the other staff:

> Rebecca: *You didn't really have a choice. I suppose it is easier just to go along and just get on, plod along, isn't it really?*
> Jenny: *Too easy!*

There were times when the co-researchers needed support regarding collaboration with doctors. When the clinical director of the DSU joined one of the meetings, I suddenly became aware that only I was talking. The co-researchers had altered their behaviour and fallen silent. I hoped that they did not feel intimidated and encouraged them to contribute their own perceptions.

On another occasion, at a planning meeting, we discussed the distribution of the questionnaires:

> Loretta: *I would just like to know when you think it would be appropriate to send these out; when would you like to distribute them?*
> Rebecca: *I personally think we should give them to our colleagues as soon as possible, but it would be nicer if the ones to the consultants came from you.*
> Loretta: *But why?*
> Jenny: *Well, we're not very important are we? They may not fill the forms in.*

The clinical director of the DSU also experienced powerlessness. Within her dual role, that of consultant anaesthetist and manager, she had initially enhanced the co-researchers' motivation for change. Yet, her commitment to the study resulted in conflict. She too experienced what could be termed the oppressive culture of the organisation.

> Loretta (at the TM's interview): *Nina said today that A. [Clinical Director] had said to her that she really wanted to improve the paediatric provision.*
> Theatre Manager (TM): *I know she does. I still can't work out why it was so dangerous for - it was felt to be a danger. [pause] This is not an hysterical woman having a turn; she felt this very, very deeply ... then the rug was pulled out from under our feet.*

Allan (1999) has highlighted senior doctors' inability to challenge a Trust's management:

> Dr B. expressed anger that his generation of senior doctors were unable to challenge the trust management, and had been disempowered. He offered an example of how power had moved, as he saw it, from doctors to managers appointed as 'political pawns'. Consultants, like himself, used that power informally and reached decisions through networks like the senior dining room. (Allan 1997, 462)

The clinical director's personal values and beliefs also appeared to be in conflict with many of her medical colleagues, particularly the surgeons. Indeed, at one of the meetings, she had openly stated her perceptions of the surgeons' lack of insight into paediatric provision:

> Clinical director: *I think that on the whole they don't care twopence really as long as they get their caseload through.*

Her view was generally reinforced by the co-researchers' informal explorations of doctors' views as well as the questionnaire results, which supported the status quo. She said to me (outside of the co-researcher meeting) that she wished to be supportive of nursing as well as medical research. According to her, some medical colleagues did not share her view; they could not see any benefits. I reflected on whose interests were being served by retaining the status quo, those of patients/users or medical staff?

There was an interesting response from an anaesthetist:

> Nina: *I spoke to J.; he is consultant anaesthetist for Mr K. He wasn't happy, only because he said it was boring. He said it gets boring only doing children!*
> Chris: *Once all the surgeons start discussing it, they could surely work out who likes doing paeds; they could alternate.*
> Loretta: *The assumption is that they all talk to each other.*
> Nina: *Get on!* [much laughter]

Not only did a large proportion of medical staff have no real desire to change, the new nursing manager of the DSU appeared to reinforce the status quo culture. There was no support or encouragement to change in the pursuit of good practice. The retiring DSU manager (A) had appeared to maintain the status quo and resisted change. The co-researchers and I hoped that the newly appointed manager (B) would adopt a more positive view towards innovation. However, her style of leadership did not appear to be any different from that of her predecessor. Conway (1996) in her description of the evolution of nursing expertise described the Traditionalist in terms of 'survival'.

> These experts were preoccupied with 'getting the work done' and managing care with scarce resources. In carrying out a task, care had a medical focus and the nurses operated as overseers and doctors' assistants. Management and doctors were perceived as all powerful. They did not value their own practice and saw themselves as powerless in terms of influence. They saw education as an optional extra and not as central to practice development. Value was attached to 'doing' and not 'reflecting'. They showed that 'papering-over-the-cracks' was what nursing was about and this others also learned to do. The dispossessed dispossessed others. (Conway 1996, 77)

Nina, the DSU nurse lecturer, had decided to leave. Loretta (to the TM at the evaluation interview):

> Nina has tried her best, but she has had enough. She has tried to establish a good working relationship with B., but, as with A., she is just not valued. She sets up all these education sessions, and without support from B. no one comes. Hopefully, I haven't made any derogatory remarks about B. [to the co-researchers], but I have told the co-researchers that I have found it difficult to work with her, and I don't normally have problems like that.

New ways of working were needed to improve the quality of service provision.

> Rebecca: A lot of what has been developed - it is not the workers who are asked, it's all above the working level.

In the change process the need to establish trust amongst health-care staff is evident. Lack of trust is partly derived from negative power

(Handy 1985), which may be seen at all levels of an organisation. Negative power is the ability to filter or distort information, instructions or requests from one part of the organisation to another. Handy refers to the use of negative power at times of low morale, irritation, stress or frustration at the failure of other influence attempts. His perspective complements the assertion by Forester (1983, 238) on the importance of applying critical theory to organisations, in order: 'To alert us to the subtle and possibly systematic ways in which social action and social actors, may be deceived, misled, manipulated, or mystified.'

Two examples reflect these disempowering processes. At one of the co-researcher meetings Chris considered:

> *If the box* [for collection of questionnaires] *was left out all the time, if you really did not want to have it* [the dedicated day], *somebody could rifle through all the ones that were positive, they could pull out those forms and throw them away.*

Equally significant was the conversation that transpired between myself and the TM, at the evaluation interview. We were exploring patient/user involvement, and I reminded her of her clear advice: *not to elicit patients' views at this time.*

> Loretta: *I mean the other evidence we don't have is from the patients themselves, and they* [the co-researchers] *were disappointed that we couldn't take that forward.*
> TM: *Well, we don't know that we can't ... it still doesn't make sense to me why it was so sensitive.*

Other power issues reflected the need for anonymity amongst some of the DSU staff who completed the questionnaire. This requirement quite surprised the co-researchers. We had agreed that all the questionnaires would be anonymous. However, in my absence (on leave), before the questionnaires were distributed, Nina suggested that they number them. Nina had used questionnaires in her post-graduate research study, and she felt that numbering would be an expedient approach. Williams (1995) cautions that maintaining confidentiality is not only a function of awareness of power as an aspect of all relationships, but it is also associated with the multiple agendas held by the researchers.

Rebecca: *They got up in arms about the numbering.*

Nina: *And I am sorry that it was my idea to number the questionnaires ... I can't believe that people felt so threatened about the number on a piece of paper.*

Loretta: *People do think now: What is going to happen to this? Is someone else going to read it and look at it? Is it going to management, and are there going to be reprisals for what I've written? It is difficult, I know, but we did put 'anonymous' on the front of the question- naire.*

Rebecca: *I think the ones that were insulted peeled the numbers off ... I was really upset about that, Nina.*

Nina: *We have certainly learnt from this.*

Process outcomes

Although the second study encompassed six months only (whereas the first study lasted fifteen months), process outcomes for the co-researchers and the TM could clearly be explicated from the group meetings and evaluation interviews. An interview proforma similar to the one in the first study was used as a prompt for the co-researchers (table 10.4).

Table 10.4: Co-researcher interview proforma.

1. How did you feel at the start of the project?
2. How has the study helped you, both professionally and personally?
3. How has the study hindered you, both personally and professionally?
4. How do you feel about the project to date?
5. How would you now like to proceed?

Participating in the study and challenging the status quo gave the co-researchers the opportunity for personal growth. They collaborated by sharing their ideas, valuing each other's contributions and those of their peers:

Rebecca: *I suppose I am looking at things differently now. I don't just have my opinion and stick to it; I do try and listen and realise you can get ideas from everybody.*

Jenny: *Yes, it made me open my eyes a bit more. I think more now and voice my opinion more now too.*

In spite of working in an oppressive culture, they did feel empowered:

> Nina: *I think the thing is everybody has grown with it. To begin with you were not sure what was going on really, and it was interesting to see how people took owner-ship of it, controlled it, did their bit. It is nice to see that rather than some academic coming in from outside and imposing their study on people.*

The co-researchers were enlightened by and felt positive about the process:

> Nina: *I think it is a good lesson for people to learn how hard it is to do this research, because of all the other factors ... I think it was nice to do, even though we don't feel there is going to be a change. It is nice to do something that really is beneficial to patients, because it is easy to do something that only affects nurses or things that you can control a bit more. We knew that we didn't have control over this and that somebody else ultimately was going to make the decisions, but it was nice to have a go - to do it. Even though maybe lots of people still feel that it couldn't work, it has raised awareness of issues.*

The following statements reflect a felt or emotional power and a perception of themselves as potential (informal) leaders:

> Chris: *Even though nothing may come of it now, I think, if in the long run it can go higher, then you can be proud that you have initiated it; you can really feel proud to be a part of that team.*
> Nina: *Others might start to think: 'Oh this is actually quite a good idea.' Snowballing - you have to have a small beginning sometimes. A lot of the time it's much easier for people to say no to something before they have really thought it through.*
> Rebecca: *There was a purpose for us in what we were doing. It wasn't just you coming in Loretta and wasting our time!* [laughter] *There is more to it. We are being pioneers.*

Stringer (1996) identifies pride/feelings of self-worth as the most important quality indicator in an action research study. It is also evident that the co-researchers have begun to personally question and openly challenge the social norms of the DSU and the power of doctors and managers. This addresses the concern of Habermas (1976) regarding whether social norms that claim legitimacy are genuinely accepted by those that follow and internalise them. Informal leadership, as exemplified in this study, should now be considered necessary for cultural change. Bate (1994, 238) believes that a radical rethink is needed to challenge 'the men- [women-] in-grey-suits brigade, the product of narrow and oppressive twentieth-century rationalist philosophies'.

The co-researchers also started to appreciate the need to update their reading. Although I kept the reading material to an absolute minimum, only Nina had read the literature that I had provided.

> Loretta: *So I've photocopied the WHO information and highlighted just a couple of paragraphs - that's all you have to read!*

Towards the end of the study my continued emphasis on reading appeared to have an impact:

> Rebecca: *As we have very few* [operating] *lists today, we have asked if we can visit the library to get some articles.*

Overall, there was no overt resentment regarding the questionnaire response by medical staff. They shared enlightened views:

> Rebecca: *I was quite pleasantly surprised how much detail was provided* [in the questionnaire] *by some of the medical staff. The comments were more thoughtful and responsible, not dismissive. That was encouraging. Most of the ones that didn't agree still put in an effort to explain why.*
>
> Chris: *I suppose in a way that is understandable, because it is probably more difficult for them to reorganise their work.*

The co-researchers' process outcomes are delineated in table 10.5.

Table 10.5: Co-researcher process outcomes (second study).

The co-researchers' process outcomes

Enlightenment
Engaging in collaborative practice
Recognition of 'small beginnings'
Insight into medical and management perspectives

Education
Reading awareness
Developing knowledge of research and change

Empowerment
'Felt' power
Ownership of project
Personal and team pride
Raised awareness of issues for peers

Emancipation
Informal leaders
Pioneering spirit
Being considered able to initiate patient-focused change

These process outcomes are similar to the outcomes that were identified for the co-researchers in the first study (see pages 149–150). From reviewing the outcomes of both studies it appears that participating in a critical action research study enables personal and group enlightenment, education and empowerment. The recognition of emancipatory practice is also clearly evident.

Process outcomes could also be explicated for the TM (see table 10.6). She too was enlightened by the action research process. She was also impressed by the enthusiasm of the DSU staff who were present at the feedback meeting:

> TM: *They started to debate between them not just with you but actually between themselves. For me that seemed a good thing to get them talking together about nursing ... what I would want is that that process continues, that these people are sort of guided to go for things that make a direct difference.*

She reflected on how the study had raised awareness of current and future education/practice development needs for the DSU nursing staff but commented:

The sad thing about that sort of gain is that it is so intan-
gible that you can't measure it.

Table 10.6: The TM's process outcomes.

The Process Outcomes of the Theatre Manager
• Recognition of the potential of empowering strategies for the DSU staff
• Valuing DSU staff's enthusiastic and creative ideas
• Valuing of the action research process
• Awareness of DSU staff's education/practice development needs
• Exploration of the organisational culture
• Recognition of qualitative outcomes

Talking and thinking deeply about nursing in the clinical setting was a new experience for the nurses in both action research studies. In her editorial on thinking about nursing futures Street (1997) states that thinking requires time and commitment: it demands a capacity to live with tensions, contradictions, ambiguities and not to foreclose on irregularities and loose ends. She believes that thinking is neither fashionable nor visible. Its products are not always evident except for the thinker and those who have been touched by thoughtful nurses and thoughtful scholarship. The TM had certainly been touched by her nurses:

Some of the things that came up were genuinely quite
interesting and actually things I hadn't thought about ...
I've had my eyes opened.

There are nurses working in the clinical setting whose qualities and commitment impress those who work with them. Greenwood (1997) suggests that the nurturing of these nurses might be preparing the leaders of tomorrow. Yet, as well as her recognising the need to both educate and nurture her staff, the TM also needed to try to decipher why the decision to support the study had changed. Reflections on the organisational culture led her to exclaim:

It's just a perfect example of how political agendas get
in the way of real achievement ... I go to a meeting, and
I think for God's sake someone just tell me what we are
talking about here because there are six different
agendas here, only one of which I understand ... I am
trying to untangle it.

As early as 1943 a paper written by Lewin refers to organisational fear and insecurity:

> Each section of the organisation usually shows some suspicion as a result of its particular type of insecurity; each section is afraid that its power or influence may be affected or that some unpleasant data be uncovered by the research. (Cartwright 1963)

Although more than half a century has elapsed since Lewin's perceptive insight, it still appears to demonstrate the culture that currently exists within many healthcare settings.

Comparisons could be made between the outcomes from the TM and those of her contemporary in the first study, the nurse unit manager (NUM). While the second study had not progressed beyond the unfreezing stage, some significant comparisons could still be made. In the first study the key themes that emerged were ongoing support, relinquishing control, conflicting loyalties, identifying positive outcomes, enhanced value and respect for staff, and an eye opener (page 163). These themes were equally relevant in the second study.

Both the managers were newly appointed as the studies commenced. It was evident that they both provided ongoing support for the study, albeit at a distance. Whereas in the first study this was an appropriate strategy, in the second study a more overt commitment by the TM may have led to a more positive response from the DSU manager. Conflicting priorities regarding financial resources presented a dilemma for the NUM. This did not appear to be a problem for the TM, who was more confused and frustrated than ethically challenged by organisational processes. Both managers could very clearly identify positive outcomes for their staff and for themselves. The NUM also articulated the positive outcomes for patients/users and other trust staff. The creative ideas that their staff had generated was an 'eye opener' for both managers (see pages 138 and 231). The recognition by both managers of their staff's value and worth should contribute to the future promotion of empowering strategies and innovative patient-focused practice.

Moving forward - framework for nurse-led change and development

While appreciating that every action research study is unique (see page 163), from the research evidence a conceptual framework regarding nurse-led change and development in clinical practice is proposed (see table 10.7). The conceptual framework was explicated from analysis of all the process and outcome data of the two studies as well as the supporting literature.

Table 10.7: A conceptual framework for nurse-led change and development in clinical practice.

Collaborative Change Agents	Change Process Strategies	Anticipated Outcomes
Insider or Outsider Facilitator and Nurses Patients/Carers Healthcare Team	Participative Facilitation	1) Nurse-led, patient-focused creative change and development Initiatives
	Personal Enhancement	
	Demonstrable Interpersonal Support	2) Personal, professional practice development
	Disempowerment Recognition	
	Staff Empowerment	

The conceptual framework may appear simplistic, but it attempts to reflect the need to address the complex socio-cultural, political and psychological factors within a healthcare setting that are evident within the clinical change process identified in the two studies. It may offer nurses, nurse managers and nurse educators an enhanced or complementary perspective regarding clinical change management. Fundamental to the development of the framework is an eclectic knowledge-base of critical social theory, change theories, collaboration, empowerment, effective leadership, clinical facilitation, reflective practice, practice development and evidence-based practice, encompassed within a systematic critical action research approach.

Chapter 11
Moving forward

'Clearly those who "are prepared to try" need managerial support and strategic vision, at all levels of the hierarchy, to implement research-based practice. It is no longer good enough to assume that individual practitioners will work in isolation, a coherent strategy which supports research and development in its widest sense is required to move this agenda forward.' (Le May et al. 1998)

Action researcher reflexivity

Action researchers need to 'put themselves on the line' (Webb 1991) to enable others to judge the quality of the research. Such reflexivity is essential if the evidence they collect is to be credible (Sapsford and Abbott 1992). Nurse-led change and development was a process of comparing risks and benefits, making individual and collective choices but mostly the realisation of a personal philosophy reflecting the assertion by McNiff (1988) that you have a responsibility to your own ideals to follow them through and convert them into reality.

I believe that:

- learning is most meaningful when it occurs in clinical practice
- clinical practitioners have a wealth of practical knowledge that is of equal value to theoretical knowledge
- the sharing of knowledge between practitioners, lecturers, managers and the healthcare team will enhance patient care, student learning, continuous professional development, reduce the theory-practice 'gap' and develop nursing knowledge
- in recognition of and to advance practitioners' clinical expertise and professional judgement they should be empowered to make changes, which they will be able to demonstrate will improve the quality of patient care

The choice of a critical action research approach, I hoped, would advance these beliefs - I wanted the study to be meaningful for the practitioners, beneficial for patients and an attempt to advance nursing knowledge. The action researcher and co-researchers function in both powerful and powerless roles. By facilitating and engaging practitioners in a self-determination strategy, I enhanced their ability to challenge structured processes of social control and decision-making and attempted to change the status quo.

Most of the time I felt that I was researching in the dark. I had no idea how the concept of co-researcher, or the extent to which a bottom-up planned change strategy, would be perceived. In my role as an outsider (in the second study), these issues appeared even more daunting. My personal experiences and perceptions are congruent with the themes of the nurse-led framework for change and development (table 10.7), i.e. participative facilitation, staff empowerment, demonstrable interpersonal support, disempowerment recognition and personal enhancement.

Participative facilitation

Facilitating the change process was a most worthwhile, if at times disquieting, experience. As I was known to the co-researchers in the first study, facilitation primarily encompassed promoting confidence and positive anticipation throughout the process of change. This is demonstrated on pages 155–157.

As a participative research facilitator in the second study I was able to engage with the co-researchers and enable a deeper consideration of perceived DSU issues and problems. However, the open dialogue that I tried to promote no doubt disturbed a carefully controlled social environment. It also appeared to have disturbed micro-political alignments and challenged individual positions of power and influence. As an outsider my initial entry into the organisation reflected Stringer's (1996) advice, to be 'as "soft" as possible'. The approach to managers, the Ethics Committee and my engagement with DSU staff was candid and non-confrontational.

Facilitating the first meeting with the co-researchers resulted in a positive outcome. While I felt disadvantaged as an outsider, I also recognised that this was advantageous in establishing a rapport with the co-researchers. By my requesting knowledge of the organisation and of the DSU, I enabled the co-researchers to share factual information as well as their personal insights. This strategy began the process of collaborative practice, particularly as two of the co-researchers had not previously met. It was reassuring to have facilitated a consensus on a key issue by the second meeting. However, I often reflected on whether I should have facilitated foreclosure quite so early in the study. The identification of a less controversial issue may have reduced my apprehension, which was increasingly evident throughout the study. Also, as the potential for conflict increased, so did my concern for the co-researchers' well-being.

The ethical dilemma for me was whether by continuing to facilitate the study I was placing the co-researchers at increasing risk of harm. With each subsequent meeting the issue of a dedicated day for children was becoming more controversial. I was concerned for the co-researchers' well-being. Was the study jeopardising their working relationships, especially with the DSU manager? The co-researchers had the right to choose whether to continue to participate in the study. Indeed, this was the ongoing informed-consent agreement. I could walk away from the organisation at any time, but could I risk the co-researchers being labelled as reprobates? What I had imagined might happen in the first study - being viewed by others as problematic and divisive - was potentially becoming a reality in the second study. While most of the time I sustained an outward appearance of calm, I needed regular reassurance from the co-researchers that all was well:

> Rebecca: *No, I didn't get any personal flak at all.*
> Loretta: *That's good. As you know, that's my constant worry.*

When the paediatric issue became politically sensitive, my apprehension and frustration increased proportionally. I tried to engender realistic expectations:

> *It's a bit like 'Big Brother', isn't it? At times I think this, then at others I think, No, this is collaborative research! ... Hopefully it is all going to turn out well, but we don't know, and we are all in it together ... Well, it is difficult to anticipate what is going to happen, but you can't until you get the questionnaires back. If people are very negative about it - well, we'll have to live with that, won't we? It will certainly conflict with what is required from a quality perspective.*

The co-researchers often voiced what I was thinking: '*Are we being realistic?*' ... '*Are we hitting our heads against a brick wall really?*'

The literature provided me with some reassurance. Huxham (1996) believes that doubt is healthy and that it reinforces the value of the group and their continuing search for solutions. Indeed, he advises facilitators to believe in the participants and their own ability to doubt. While this advice could sustain me in the short-term, I became fully aware that the co-researchers needed to feel and be empowered to effect the change.

Staff empowerment

I often experienced apprehension regarding the development of both studies. Yet I could also recognise personal feelings of empowerment. In the first study it became evident that nurse empowerment resulted in patient empowerment (see chapter 6 'Group - Empowerment'). Also, the co-researcher evaluation (table 6.4, p. 147) demonstrated a change in power relationships particularly between nurse and patient. This outcome was empowering for me as I had initiated and participated in the change process.

To empower my colleagues I mostly led from behind, my preferred position. My strategy at meetings was therefore mainly to wait for the co-researchers to initiate action. On very few occasions did I directly ask a colleague to do something, *'Benita, you're co-ordinating the leaflets, aren't you; so could you ... ?'* I would close a meeting by stating, for example, *'Well, before we meet again, I'll type up the drug leaflets and contact Dr G.'* Co-researchers would then volunteer what they would be doing between meetings, *'I'll dig out some current info on PCA.' 'I'll ask E. [ward clerk] to photocopy the completed operation leaflets.' 'I'll clear out the old files so we can keep them all together in the ward.'* No pressure was placed on the quiet co-researchers to speak. Yet, when they did speak, it was powerful and significant as they reflected ideas that no one else had voiced, *'There should be a space for the anaesthetist's signature on the patient PCA forms to ensure they have administered the loading dose.'*

During the group meetings in both studies, I was consciously avoiding a didactic approach. Consequently, I provided very little in the way of preparatory advice or literature etc., relying instead on the co-researchers to identify their learning needs. This strategy reflected 'training follows change', one of the (six) crucial factors that Ottaway (1976 cited by Lancaster and Lancaster 1982) identifies in the change process. He advocates that, rather than trying to change people for new skills and expecting them to apply them, the participator (co-researcher) begins to feel the need for new knowledge and skill, which is then supplied. This experiential approach results from personal and group reflection and action.

In the second study, I began to feel empowered when permission to conduct the study was granted, both from the corporate level of the organisation and from the Ethics Committee. From past experience of the first study, gaining permission to undertake the study had been the most difficult process for me. Yet, in the second study, the enlightened responses from senior staff towards an outsider made me feel cautiously optimistic. However, this optimism was to be significantly challenged throughout the process of initiating bottom-up change.

In spite of my increasing unease, there were four key reasons why I continued to facilitate the change process:

- the co-researchers' shared commitment
- the evidence in the literature
- the commitment from the DSU clinical director
- the co-researchers' response to the reticence displayed by senior management

I considered all of these to be empowering experiences. Through sharing beliefs about nursing with the co-researchers, I became increasingly supportive of the proposed change. This reflects Handy's (1985) assertion that participation increases commitment if the individual considers participation worthwhile and legitimate. In spite of the political tensions, the co-researchers' personal beliefs and increasing commitment were evident, for example:

> I realise that more and more the patients should be listened to.
> We are committed to what we take on, aren't we?
> But then, at the end of the day, surely the priority should be providing a quality service?

Supporting evidence from the literature

The evidence in the literature strongly supported the second key reason for facilitating change (see above). Shared knowledge gleaned from the literature was an enlightening and empowering experience for us all. Before searching the literature neither I nor the co-researchers had appreciated that paediatric provision in DSUs had been extensively addressed. To read both government and medical reports on the issue, as well as the challenging perspectives in the nursing literature, which reinforced the innovation, was also a liberating experience.

Support from the hierarchy?

Legitimation of the initiative by the most senior member of the DSU medical staff (the clinical director) was an empowering process. This commitment, from a key stakeholder, was a significant motivator for change. I was delighted that she was so supportive of a nurse-led bottom-up initiative. She reinforced the co-researchers' perception of the lack of support for the initiative by some of the surgeons. Yet more significant was the lack of organisational support for her. It became evident that she was powerless to support the change in the short-term. Indeed, this outcome reflected the evidence in the literature (Allan 1997) regarding the potential disempowerment of senior medical staff by management.

Yet the management response, rather than frustrating and disempowering the co-researchers, enhanced their resolve for change (page 199). Interestingly, Hart and Bond (1996) identify a similar effect when senior managers responded negatively to a research project. The authors report that the unintended consequence of this crisis was to deepen the ward sisters' commitment to the project and increase their preparedness to participate as a group in trying to improve the situation. The co-researchers' reference to their perceived powerlessness by management contrasted sharply with their feelings of group empowerment:

> *They know they should have had it organised from the beginning, and it is their way of thinking, right these girls who are nothing really, because we are not part of a big team, a big establishment, we are not really anything, not management.*
> *Not in the hierarchy.*
> *And then all of a sudden we come up with this ...*
> *Yes, that's right.*
> *They look stupid.* [everyone talking at once]
> *It* [senior management's letter, see box 8.1] *is also their way of saying that they made a boob, isn't it?"* [much laughter]

While I could acknowledge the co-researchers' elation and feelings of empowerment, I could not, on this occasion, reciprocate. I was placed in a perplexing position. I could try to empathise with the co-researchers and support their view. Yet a paradox was evident as, while they felt empowered by the senior management's response, I personally felt disempowered, particularly by the letter. I could not engage with the co-researchers in a 'them versus us' scenario.

Co-researcher empowerment

Co-researcher feelings of empowerment were also evident during the fortnightly meetings. On two occasions I was delighted to be 'put in my place'. In one particular meeting it was pointed out to me that I was 'doing all the talking'! On another occasion, my views were challenged:

> You said it was a lot of hard work collecting in question-
> naires. In fact, there was no hard work, they were given
> out, people put them back in the box and there was very
> little hassle to get people to collect them.

The two-week gap between meetings caused me some anxiety especially as there appeared to be little support from the DSU manager. I wanted the co-researchers to maintain their enthusiasm for the study and to feel that they did have ongoing support, albeit from a distance. How could I reinforce the feelings of empowerment? The week following a meeting I would write to each co-researcher and, on occasions, enclose a relevant article to support the initiative. I had assumed that they would automatically read the information, but only Nina did. My exasperation eventually became evident:

> It is quite good actually, what it says. But it is quite inter-
> esting that you haven't read it or you haven't got the
> time or whatever, because you wonder why do they
> print these and who are they aimed at? It's like a lot of
> things, and I know that there is so much written infor-
> mation about, but what is the point if people don't read
> them?

This outburst led to two defensive responses - 'There is no time to read here' and 'I would find it hard to study and work full time.' This led me to reflect on the culture of the DSU and the extent to which professional reading and updating of knowledge was actively encouraged. Also, reading refereed articles and policy document summaries is a developmental process. It was interesting that this type of reading should be associated with formal studying. None of the co-researchers, besides Nina, had undertaken any further or higher education. Camiah (1997) identifies similar findings from exploring the utilisation of nursing research in practice. Nurses found research reports incomprehensible, and many of the nurses were unable to find time for studying research reports and keeping up with new developments in educational research. Wright et al.'s (1996) Australian survey of 410 medical-surgical and psychiatric nurses reveals that only 15% of respondents often read research journals.

> A challenge for those committed to improving practice
> is to motivate nurses to read and evaluate published
> research studies. (Wright et al. 1996, 18)

The co-researchers' 'reading avoidance' appeared to include all professional literature, not exclusively research reports. Towards the end of the unfreezing process they began to appreciate the importance of updating their knowledge and even initiated a visit to the library. An interesting discovery, although one I had previously considered, was that, according to the theatre manager:

> (TM, in her evaluation interview): *As far as I can ascertain, the DSU staff have received, up until now, zero development.*

Demonstrable interpersonal support

Having to switch off from clinical work at the group meetings was often difficult for the co-researchers, especially when coping with a heavy workload. Coping strategies included humour and digression. Yet on occasions, in the first study, I was the scapegoat as I was the reason for the co-researchers' additional stress, although this was never directly stated. Instead I was at times accused of being pedantic and castigated for using 'theoretical jargon'. I accepted this transference of stress and anxiety without becoming too defensive.

Meyer (1993a) refers to the action researcher's extreme isolation and self-doubt, which is aggravated by having to learn to develop methods and strategies in the field (unlike most research, which can be planned in advance). However, a mutual support strategy for myself and the day sister often occurred after the meetings. We offered each other encouragement, exchanged professional information and gossip. We often spoke of the effects of the study on the co-researchers and, in particular, how the more quiet of the nurses were 'blossoming'. Titchen (action researcher/physiotherapist) and Binnie (ward sister) (1993) caution that their partnership could become too cosy, i.e. being uncritical, unquestioning of the other's thinking and behaviour, appearing to be constantly 'in league' with one another. In retrospect this did not appear to be a problem for us: we often openly challenged one another at the group meetings. I felt that our partnership was our strength and our mutual respect and compatibility engendered confidence in one another and in the co-researchers.

In the second study, digression and humour were also the two key coping strategies identified during the group meetings. Digression ranged from exchanges regarding Christmas planning, families and holidays to microwave cooking. I actively encouraged these social exchanges over coffee, especially as there was a two-week gap between meetings:

> Loretta: *It can be very difficult to come straight off, try to unwind and then refocus on the study.*

The first study had enabled me to appreciate the importance of social exchange prior to the focus of the meeting. As an outsider in the second study I needed even more to re-engage with the group, and they with one another. We shared information regarding our social lives. This enabled me to recognise our common links, particularly that we were all working mothers. As an 'outsider' I felt more apprehensive than in the first study in my ability to re-establish the momentum for change. I was relieved that the co-researchers were often able to view the change process from a humorous perspective:

> Loretta: *That's the 'problem' with research you see.*
> Rebecca: *Well yes, we are finding that out!* [much laughter]
> Jenny: *We are probably going to be blacklisted as well* [for initiating a paediatric day]; *we'd better hide our name badges!*
> Patsy: *Don't give them out at all* [the questionnaires] *just fill them in ourselves! No I'm only joking.*
> Chris: *By the time we get all the questionnaires back and we sort things out it'll be five years.*

The continued importance of interpersonal support was equally relevant for me. I was delighted to be invited to the DSU Christmas party: Rebecca was one of the key organisers. Unfortunately, work commitments prevented me from attending, but I welcomed any opportunity to meet other members of staff. This often occurred when having coffee with Nina in the staff sitting room (before or after a co-researcher meeting).

My relationship with Nina encompassed the need for mutual support that I had experienced in the first study (with the day sister). Indeed,

Webb (1989), Meyer (1993a), and Waterman (1995) identify the need for emotional support for action researchers. Nina and I had, we discovered, much in common. We were both educationalists with a strong practice focus. We both shared similar experiences from our separate encounters with the DSU manager. We always remained behind after the co-researcher meetings to reflect on the process. Nina's insights were most enlightening, and we provided reassurance and support for one another. On the research process she said:

> It is a good time to be doing it though, because there is so much now about protocols and standards based on research involving staff ... I think it has reinforced the problems of doing research in devising a questionnaire that people understand; however hard you try to use English, plain English and constructed in a way that people can answer the questions, there are still problems with questionnaires ... I was impressed with how much people did contribute.

Nina's view as a co-researcher reflected that of the day sister in the first study. As experienced nurses they recognised the need to relinquish control to enable collaborative practice:

> Day sister: I think perhaps sometimes I find it hard to devolve things to others, but I do try.
> Nina: I think that sometimes it is difficult not to take over too much. I felt that sometimes I was taking over, and I shouldn't have.

Nina enabled me to validate my views of the oppressive culture within the DSU and the organisation. I sometimes felt that whenever we moved one step forward we were then compelled to take three steps back! This was particularly so when we asked for questionnaire feedback. The telephone calls (pages 194 and 195) left me feeling unsupported. This was especially regarding the response from the TM, implying that the Audit Department's comments could negate the study. Also, the letter from senior management (box 8.1) appeared to me to renege on their initial agreement to support the study. Being *advised* to withhold the patients' questionnaire was yet another compounding factor. I knew that I would not be party to 'privileged information' but was grateful when the TM in her evaluation interview alluded to these issues:

You had a whole cocktail of influences, nothing to do
with the project, that directly affected it.

Although feelings of empowerment were apparent throughout the
study, there were equally significant disempowering experiences.

Disempowerment recognition

The most challenging issues for me were those that reflected actual and
perceived power issues. In the first study there were problems with
medical staff, i.e. a doctor's devaluing of an experienced nurse's advice,
and co-researcher feedback avoidance. Yet positive, as opposed to
anticipated negative, feedback was received from senior medical staff,
e.g. the consultant anaesthetist's agreement to PCA and the letter
regarding PSM (box 5.1). In the first study, I felt disempowered by the
initial refusal by the district general manager and the Ethics
Committee to commence the study (page 69).

In the second study I knew that, as an outsider, I was potentially
disadvantaged before the study commenced. My knowledge deficits
included no prior knowledge of the DSU or of the hospital that I was to
enter. In agreement with the director of patient services I delayed the
start of the study until the new TM was in post. It was then I was told
that a new DSU manager was to be appointed. I could only hope, in
retrospect somewhat naïvely, that the new appointee would welcome a
collaborative study and eventually become involved in innovative
change. I knew that the new managers would both need to establish
their power-base and develop their working relationship. I hoped that
they both valued or would come to value new ways of working. I also
identified one common factor - none of us had any direct insight into
the culture of the organisation.

I shared my perception of collaboration with both managers. I
explained that I recognised that the study might not be high on their
list of priorities (even though I wanted it to be). I maintained the
profile of the study by ongoing communication with the managers both
verbally and in writing. The TM was positive and supportive, albeit
from a distance. This reflected my experience in the first study; the unit
manager was also new in post and my first acquaintance with her was as
I commenced the study. The polite indifference that I experienced
from the DSU manager was the complete reversal of the support and
participation of her contemporary (the ward sister) in the first study.
Her distancing from myself and, it appeared, the co-researchers was for
me a constant source of anguish and concern and felt disempowering. I
hoped that I could demonstrate to her that I was facilitating a process

that possibly challenged her nursing values but not her power-base and authority.

There were a number of instances that reflected disempowerment. One example occurred every fortnight. Trying to create a psychologically safe environment for the co-researchers was difficult when there was no specific room for meetings. Each time I arrived at the DSU I had to re-negotiate with the manager a site for our meeting. We had previously agreed and recorded in the DSU diary the dates and times of all of the fortnightly meetings. Yet on no occasion was a room identified for the meeting. I found this process frustrating and at times considered it obstructive. This was especially as I had observed both the manager and her efficient secretary respond instantly to long-term requests by other visitors (doctors) for access to the DSU. On one occasion we were told to hold the meeting in the reception area where there were newly admitted patients. I had to tactfully remind the manager of the difficulties of maintaining confidentiality especially regarding the 'sensitive' issue that we were discussing. Nevertheless I still hoped for improvement:

> Loretta [fifth meeting, opening remark]: *I've just spoken to B., and she said that she might be able to join us towards the end of the meeting.*

I admitted my defeat to the co-researchers at the evaluation group interview:

> *I try to link to B., but I felt there was a block, which I couldn't get through ... I did say please come for half the meeting or ten minutes' update, but she didn't physically come so there wasn't that support, and I felt that all the way along, which I find quite upsetting in a way because her members of staff were trying to do something to improve the care of patients in her unit.*

I was also disappointed that she did not join the TM at the feedback session to the DSU staff (although she was on duty).

> Loretta (to the TM): *How useful it would have been if she could have joined us, because, whatever she was feeling, we could have explored it.*

I acknowledged her traditional management style, which was primarily reflected in the need to accommodate the wishes of the medical staff. Greenwood (1997), in her exploration of leadership and change, provides a classic example of the power-coercive ward sister:

> Rules and policies were meant to be followed to the letter without question. She was demanding of her staff and rarely seemed supportive. She ... effectively undermined and disempowered people. (Greenwood 1997, 24)

I discovered at the TM's evaluation interview that the DSU manager was undertaking a trial period. The person who was to have been appointed to the re-advertised post had declined to take up the position at the eleventh hour. Consequently, the current DSU manager's position was tenuous. This information made me initially reconsider my perception of her. Had I been too judgmental too soon? She must have known that she was a second choice. However, I concluded that my analysis of her behaviour was justified. If she had been dynamic and forward-thinking, the words used by the TM to describe the first applicant, she would have at least considered the innovation. Also, I wondered why she had not reconsidered her resistant stance when it became evident that this was not shared by either her senior manager nor the director of the DSU.

Overall, the TM recognised the potential for disempowerment, particularly in relation to time constraints, power conflicts and feedback avoidance:

> The timing was very bad for you, although I realise that you had already delayed the start. You got two new managers who didn't know each other.

I felt hopeful that the TM would start to lead on some of the developments that had been identified from the DSU feedback meeting (pages 213–214). Indeed, since taking up her post, she had identified two weak links in the organisation:

> This trust in general has extremely good staff, although often not in key positions. There is a whole layer of very good, solid, reliable, imaginative staff. Unfortunately, the weakest level currently is the management level below me ... Apparently, the medical staff have a very poor track record here of joining in and attending meetings, particularly the general surgeons.

The disempowering culture of the organisation was reflected in the study. The effect was evident within Nina's observation:

> *I am sorry that it was my idea to number the question-naires; I was surprised that people felt so threatened about that number on a piece of paper - but you learn from it.*

What had I learnt? Anticipation of and recognition of disempowering processes must be explored. Indeed, this reflects a critical social theory approach. Adopting the critical action research approach enables a collaborative way of challenging the status quo and effecting change. Yet, in this hospital, I felt that I had facilitated the unfreezing of just the tip of the iceberg.

Personal enhancement

Personal enhancement occurred through collaboration. I felt reassured that even as an outsider I was able to share my beliefs about nursing, acquire new knowledge from the co-researchers and the literature, and engage in group problem-solving. I recognised that I could create a psychologically safe environment for the exchange of ideas and start to establish trust. This was in spite of an organisational culture, in the second study, which I considered to be disempowering.

My belief in collaborative practice has been reinforced, especially between practitioners, educators and managers. In the first study, I participated in innovation and change in, what I hoped, was a non-threatening manner. I acquired insight into areas for future development, especially for cultivating mutually collaborative strategies with peers, medical staff and other members of the multi-professional team, for joint decision-making and practice. I gained personal satisfaction both from enhancing the quality of surgical nursing care and from the surgical nurses' personal and professional development. For the future I hoped that the co-researchers would now value group problem-solving and, where appropriate, initiate, implement and evaluate change.

In the second study, personal enhancement was also derived from the recognition of personal perceptions of negative feedback and assumptions. I have previously alluded to the unanticipated response by the co-researchers to the letter from senior management (box 8.1). I had assumed that the co-researchers would have felt, like me, demoralised and disempowered. Yet the opposite occurred. Their response was for them cathartic and liberating.

Another assumption of mine, which was also severely challenged, was that the manager of the DSU would eventually contribute to the study. When she made it evident that she was opposed to the innovation, I initially assumed that the study would be terminated. The literature reinforced my belief regarding the contribution of this key stakeholder. Between 1980 and 1985 a number of research studies on the role of the ward sister were completed (Pembrey 1980, Orton 1981, Fretwell 1982, 1985, Marson 1982, Ogier 1982, 1986, 1989, Alexander 1983, Farnish 1983, Runciman 1983 and Lathlean and Farnish 1984). The most outstanding finding that emerged from the studies was the power of the ward sister. She was the key figure in the organisation, was a role model for the staff and created the ward learning climate (Cameron-Buccheri and Ogier 1994).

Yet, once again, the opposite occurred. In spite of her resistance to change, the need to pursue the initiative was reinforced by her senior, the TM, and the medical director of the DSU. My journal records my ongoing frustration. I hoped that she was a 'late adopter' and that she would eventually recognise the need for change. It seemed to me that, as the literature suggests (Roberts 1997), she appeared to suppress her nursing values or, indeed, needed to regain them.

In the first study the NUM recognised the dilemma of conflicting professional and bureaucratic values. In spite of financial restrictions, she chose not to compromise her professional values (page 135). The outcome of her risk assessment was positive for the patients (PCA). Yet, in the second study, even if the DSU manager had been supportive of the initiative and not compromised her nursing values the outcome would have been the same, i.e. the letter from senior management (box 8.1). I had assumed that a telephone conversation with the nurse director of patient services (page 171) plus a follow-up letter had secured support for the study. I was unable to contact her to renegotiate support, because she was on long-term sick leave. I considered whether O'Kelly's (1994) observation regarding the marginalisation of nurse leaders at a senior level was apparent in this hospital trust. This could have been one of the key issues within 'the cocktail of influences' that impinged on the study, alluded to by the TM (page 244).

The insight that I have acquired from these experiences has been always to explore my own assumptions. This may not be perceived as a significant conclusion. Yet this conclusion reflects the importance, when attempting to enact a critical social theory approach, not only of trying to identify and challenge the underlying assumptions of the status quo, but also of continually challenging one's own personal assumptions throughout the study.

One assumption of mine that was reinforced was the non-use of reflective journals by the co-researchers. I based my view on the outcome of the first study and the limited reading that was evident throughout the second study. In the first study I imposed the journals on the co-researchers and realised too late that this was not collaborative practice. In the second study I explored the purpose of reflection and stated that the use of a journal was entirely voluntary. The notebooks were issued prior to distribution of the questionnaires. I was delighted by the 100% positive uptake.

> *Write down whatever you want. For example - how you feel, what colleagues say to you, what was straightforward, any problems ...*
> *Good idea actually.*
> *They are your own property. I won't ask to read them or anything. Just bring them to the meeting and whatever is there you may wish to share.*
> *Goes in my top pocket.*

While I believed that the journals would provide personal enhancement and understanding, the co-researchers (at the evaluation interview) did not feel that they had anything 'important' to note or to reflect upon.

> *Did you actually write anything in your personal journals?*
> *I have asked everybody and said, 'You must have written something', but we didn't.*
> *I knew you wouldn't - isn't that interesting?*

Although, as in the first study, I had emphasised that we were sharing not judging personal reflections, even Nina, who was familiar with the reflection literature, had not undertaken the process. I had to conclude, as in the first study, that group reflection, rather than personal reflection, met the co-researchers' need for sharing and support.

A range of feelings

As I withdrew from the second study I experienced a sense of loss, which still remains. I felt that I had not completed what I had hoped to achieve. In spite of the problems that emerged, I had, in particular, valued the co-researcher meetings. From the group evaluation interview, I was overwhelmed, as in the first study, by the co-researchers' personal reflections on the outcomes of, what seemed for me, a relatively brief encounter. Also, the co-researchers felt empowered to continue their meetings; this was also an outcome of the first study. I could only hope that with the TM's support they would continue and that they would be encouraged to explore a less sensitive issue. However, I still believe that it would be highly unlikely that they would succeed at implementing any initiative (even a drinks machine) without the current DSU manager's support.

Although there were significant problems to overcome, particularly within the second study, I now feel a sense of achievement at having adopted the role of both an insider and outsider action researcher. Which did I prefer and what were the significant differences? Waterman et al. (1995) note that problems will arise whether the action researcher is an insider or an outsider. There are pros and cons for each approach, but I personally felt more disadvantaged in the second study. The key differences revolve around familiarity with the staff, the setting, the culture of the organisation and the key stakeholders.

In the second study I was a stranger with partial vision exploring an unfamiliar setting. The co-researchers opened my eyes to the setting, the culture, staff relationships and the organisation. I therefore knowingly had to place far more trust in these co-researchers than was required in the first study. Also, having no prior knowledge of the staff enabled a less judgmental perspective of their views. As an insider I knew the staff and the environment; consequently, their perspectives and behaviour were considered in relation to my past experience of working amongst them. I also began to realise that the action researcher did not have to be a known and credible facilitator, as I had assumed in the first study. I had been accepted into the organisation and the unit as an unknown outsider and felt able to initiate the facilitation process.

The most significant outcome for me from undertaking the studies has been the realisation of the potential of bottom-up change and development within a critical action research approach. While the process of change should be systematic and sensitive to the needs of stakeholders, its value and power should not be underestimated. This was clearly identified, particularly in the first study. The challenging of the structures of social control was also clearly evident in the second study, but I had not appreciated the strength of the co-researchers' commitment to change that evolved from engagement in this empowering process. The two studies reinforced for me both the practitioners' creativity and their ability to engage in collaborative research to enhance the quality of patient care. I have concluded that, while I felt more disadvantaged as an outsider, I could more fully appreciate the significance of co-researcher trustworthiness and more distant working relationships.

Stringer (1996) notes that, if it does not make a difference, in a very specific way, for practitioners and/or their clients, an action research project has failed to achieve its objectives. On reflection, of all the themes identified that of 'eye opener' was significant for us all. We not only shared our nursing values and ideas, we put them into practice, evaluated them and reflected on the process. Both senior managers were impressed by their staff's creativity and enlightened by the outcomes (see tables 6.6 and 10.6).

Guidance for critical action researchers

Waterman (1995) identifies 14 categories to demonstrate the change process for other action researchers. Her categories are power and ideology, support, ownership, motivation, education and reflection, anxieties and stress, communication networks, facilitators, research participants' roles, execution of change, physical environment, patient numbers; permanency and qualifications of staff and wider bureaucratic structures and policies. These categories are most useful and relevant and to a greater extent clearly fit within this study. However, the explication of a conceptual framework for nurse-led change and development in clinical practice (table 10.7) provides nurse action researchers with five key integrating change strategies: staff empowerment, disempowerment recognition, demonstrable interpersonal support, participative facilitation and personal enhancement. It is proposed that the likelihood of successfully implementing a change in clinical practice will be enhanced by putting these integrating strategies into practice. A formal schema is set out below:

Staff empowerment

- establish corporate and directorate agreement and secure ongoing support
- negotiate with the Ethics Committee the required action research information
- establish collaborative agreement with the ward/unit manager and medical staff

- negotiate 'protected time' and continuity of co-researcher meetings
- negotiate channels of communication to maintain continuity of information and feedback for co-researchers and staff
- ensure feedback from patients/peers/managers/multi-professional team

Disempowerment recognition

- provide verbal/written explanations for all stakeholders on the bottom-up critical action research approach, and the role of the action researcher, the co-researcher, the stakeholder
- identify and explore power issues and conflict resolution
- acknowledge that patients' needs have precedence over co-researcher participation at group meetings

Demonstrable interpersonal support

- provide continuous support through open communication
- create opportunities to enable shared values
- share and explore supporting evidence for change from, for example
  - group reflection on practice
  - stakeholder perceptions (patients/peers/multi-professional team)
  - national and local policies
  - professional literature
  - research studies
  - past personal experiences

- acknowledge that change often takes longer than anticipated
- undertake ongoing risk assessment of the innovation with the co-researchers
- appreciate humorous diversion and digression
- ensure continuous support from all levels of management

Participative facilitation

- be familiar with the action research, change and critical social science literature
- enlist ward/unit manager's ongoing support and participation
- negotiate an appropriate environment for group meetings
- explore the organisational culture in regard to:
  - practice development
  - innovative change
  - patient/user involvement
  - intraprofessional and multi-professional collaboration
  - senior management ongoing support

- ensure co-researcher initial and ongoing consent to participate
- define the roles of the action researcher/facilitator and co-researcher
- value each co-researcher's contribution
- encourage exploration of patient-focused problems/issues
- establish group consensus/negotiated agreement for identified change
- enlist multi-professional co-operation and collaboration
- establish ongoing action plans within tentative time frames
- ensure the identification of empowering and disempowering processes
- undertake process and outcome evaluations
- co-ordinate collaborative report writing

Personal enhancement

- encourage a voluntary approach for co-researcher self-selection and participation
- support the emergence of each co-researcher's felt need for information and professional development
- as the action researcher/facilitator, ensure personal professional support throughout the change process
- recognise that the role of the action researcher encompasses that of co-participant, co-learner, stakeholder, as well as facilitator.

The key aim for the critical action researcher is to reconcile the tension between the espoused goals of democracy and emancipation with the complexities of power and oppression (Jennings and Graham in Zuber-Skerritt 1996). The guidance above provided within the nurse-led change and development framework (table 10.7) offers one approach for achieving this aim.

The future

Undertaking critical action research has been an enlightening process, which has permeated my personal and professional life. The study enabled me to explore a research approach hitherto unknown to me. Although the critical action research approach has yet to be widely recognised, understood and valued, it is proposed that it should be seriously considered when planning change and development approaches in clinical practice settings, particularly within the clinical governance (Department of Health 1998) and *Making A Difference* (Department of Health 1999) agendas.

Support for, and routine application of, evidence-based practice into everyday work are central to the clinical governance agenda

(Department of Health 1998). Nursing literature identifies the difficulty practitioners may have in critically appraising research and particularly in utilising evidence for practice in their own clinical area (Mulhall and Le May 2001). A recent nurse-led critical action research study, in a Recovery ward within an NHS Trust hospital, started to address these issues (Bellman 2001), but the withdrawal of corporate management's ongoing support became increasingly evident:

> Recovery Sister: *But you don't empower people and then disempower them ... it's very disconcerting and quite ruthless to do that, and it isn't how you go about raising morale, standards, enhancing the quality of care. All these are the aims of the trust now and certainly come from government policy in relation to clinical governance, evidence-based practice ... so it's really mixed messages.*
> Unit Manager: *I think it's got huge potential* [the project], *but you think of collaborative working, and you think of empowering people ... bottom-up stuff ... frightening for some.*

Undertaking research within the critical paradigm has enabled me to appreciate, like Stringer (1996), that knowledge (for nurse-led change and development) is as much about politics as it is about understanding. While the government continues to advocate 'empowering frontline staff, empowering patients, and changing the culture and structure of the NHS' (Department of Health 2001, 12), the need continues for a major shift in the values, culture and leadership of the NHS (Walshe at al 2000).

However, nursing too needs to consider its culture. The 'tall poppy' syndrome identified by Faugier (1992) is often seen in nursing when individuals, and groups of individuals, who challenge and change things and stand out from the crowd, are greeted with fear, hostility and envy rather than praise and encouragement (Surman and Wright 1998). Tall poppies stand out as bold and non-conformist and are found at every level of the nursing hierarchy.

> Our tall poppies represent our maturity, our diversity and our flair as a profession. If we chop them down, we reduce nursing to a profession in which initiative goes unrewarded and being different is not encouraged. We desperately need our tall poppies, and we all need to take pride in their achievements. (Faugier 1992, 20)

The tall poppies, particularly those who are frontline/grassroots practitioners, need nurturing. They need their colleagues' recognition, support and compassion for their commitment to nurse-led change and development. Advanced nurse practitioners, i.e. those practising at a higher level, are expected to lead change and development of staff and nursing practice. Their transformational leadership skills should contribute to the facilitation and implementation of evidence-based practice. However, there may well be a need to develop collaborative clinical research skills as there is evidence that currently advanced practitioners spend very little time undertaking this aspect of their role, as research is seen as a luxury and consequently is given only lip-service (Woods 2000).

Zuber-Skerritt (1996) and Edmonstone (1995) reflect on the extensive literature on organisational innovation, quality management and change and development, which they believe is predominantly ineffective in practice. For the future an integrative organisational culture for innovative change and development and continuous quality improvement is required, which should reflect the following:

- corporate management courage and wisdom
- understanding the process of empowerment of staff, believing in it and actually doing it
- knowing how to design, lead and manage macro- and micro-organisational change and development projects
- creating transitional links between boundaries
- valuing learning and growth in the medium-term over pain avoidance, traditional benefit and ego in the short-term
- understanding that what has been taken on is not a limited organisational improvement but a new way of life

(adapted from Zuber-Skerritt 1996, 92)

In her review of the World Health Organisation's priorities for a common nursing research agenda, Hirschfeld (1998) concludes that the profession is faced with a major challenge of genuinely enabling nurses at the grassroots level to pose research questions and to receive the necessary support and education with which to actually explore issues that arise in any new encounter with a patient, a family or a community. Serious consideration should be given to the critical action research process as an effective way to achieve this change in practice. However, in the UK, a further challenge is to convince the majority of hospital managers (amongst others) of the potential of this dynamic change strategy. Zuber-Skerritt (1996) believes that more research and development work is needed to resolve the problem of dealing with people and organisations having positivist mindsets and being resistant to the notions of (critical) action research. Dadds (1998) considers that examined personal experience may be the greatest resource available for the growth of practical theory and wisdom.

Tross and Cavanagh (1996) note the many changes occurring in the NHS not just to economic and funding policies but also at the very heart of nursing care delivery. They caution that unless healthcare organisations tap into the creative potential of their employees, change and innovation will not become a reality. They even predict that staff empowered to innovate will be not only desirable but absolutely essential for the survival of the organisation. One way to address these perspectives is to engage in collaborative nurse-led change and development through the process of critical action research, which will also integrate working, learning and researching, explore the evidence for change and development, implement and evaluate patient-focused innovation, identify new knowledge for practice and achieve so much more. Engaging in the process brings a sense of achievement and enrichment to working life and a recognition of how all nurses can contribute to change and development in clinical practice.

References

Acharya S (1994) The need for a facilitator for registered nurses. Paediatric Nursing 6(4) 8-11.

Adamson B J, Kenny D T and Wilson-Barnett J (1995) The impact of perceived medical dominance on the workplace satisfaction of Australian and British nurses. Journal of Advanced Nursing 21, 172-183.

Aggleton P and Chalmers H (1985) Models and theories 6: Roper's activities of living model. Nursing Times 81, 59-61 (February 13).

Aggleton P and Chalmers H (1986) Nursing Models and the Nursing Process. Basingstoke: Macmillan Education.

Aggleton P and Chalmers H (2000) Nursing Models and Nursing Practice (second edition). Basingstoke: Macmillan.

Alexander M F (1983) Learning to Nurse: Integrating Theory and Practice Edinburgh: Churchill Livingstone.

Alfaro-LeFevre R (1998) Applying Nursing Process: a step-by-step guide (fourth edition). Philadelphia: Lippincott.

Allan H (1997) Reflexivity: A comment on feminist ethnography. NT research 2(6), 455-467.

Allen D G (1985) Nursing research and social control: alternative models of science that emphasise understanding and emancipation. Image: The Journal of Nursing Scholarship 17, 58-64.

Allen J (1996) Between the trapezes - making the most of change. Journal of Nursing Management 4, 39-43.

Allen C V (1997) Nursing Process in Collaborative Practice. Stamford, Connecticut: Appleton and Lange.

Allsop J (1984) Health Policy in the NHS. London: Longman.

Alvesson M and Willmott M (1996) Making Sense of Management. London: Sage.

Andrews-Evans M (1997) The leadership challenge in nursing. Nursing Management 4(5), 8-11.

Argyris C (1980) Inner Contradictions of Rigorous Research. New York: Academic Press.

Argyris C and Schon D (1974) Theory in Practice. San Francisco: Jossey Bass.

Asbridge J (2001) Share deal. Nursing Standard 15(17), 17-18.

Ashcroft K and Griffiths M (1989) Reflective Teachers and Reflective Tutors: school experience in an initial teacher education course. Journal of Education for Teaching 15(1), 35-52.

Aspland T, Macpherson I, Proudford C and Whitmore L (1996) Critical collaborative action research as a means of curriculum inquiry and empowerment. Educational Action Researcher 4(1), 93-104.

Astedt-Kurki P and Liukkonen A (1994) Humour in nursing care. Journal of Advanced Nursing 20, 183-188.

Atkins S and Murphy K (1993) Reflection: a review of the literature. Journal of Advanced Nursing 18, 1188-1192.

Atwell J D, Burn J M B, Dewar A K and Freeman N V (1997) Paediatric day-case surgery. The Journal of One Day Surgery. Autumn, 6-8.

Audit Commission (1990) A short cut to better services: day surgery in England and Wales. London: HMSO.

Audit Commission (1991) The Virtue of Patients: Making the Best Use of Ward Nursing Resources. London: HMSO.

Audit Commission (1997) Anaesthesia Under Examination. London: HMSO.

Baillie L (1994) Nurse teachers' feelings about participating in clinical practice: an exploratory study. Journal of Advanced Nursing 20, 150-159.

Baker H, and Pearson A (1993) Care or self-care? Self-administration of medication in hospital? Journal of Clinical Nursing 2, 251-255.

Bartunek J M and Louis M R (1996) Insider/Outsider Team Research. Qualitative Research Methods Series 40. California: Sage.

Bate P (1994) Strategies for Cultural Change. Oxford: Butterworth Heinemann.

Becker M H and Maiman L A (1975) Sociobehavioural determinants of compliance with health and medical care recommendations. Medical Care 13(1).

Bellman L (1989) Nurses' attitudes towards nursing care plans. BSc (Hons) Nursing Studies Dissertation, University of Surrey, Guildford.

Bellman L (1993) Nurses' attitudes towards the use of nursing care plans. Journal of Clinical Nursing 2(4).

Bellman L (1994) Principles of educating patients. Surgical Nurse 7(1), 7-10.

Bellman L (1996) Changing nursing practice through reflection on the Roper, Logan and Tierney model: the enhancement approach to action research. Journal of Advanced Nursing 24, 129-138.

Bellman L (1997) 'Do not believe a word that I say': a critical science approach to advancing nursing practice. Managing Clinical Nursing 1(2), 70-74.

Bellman L (1999) Nurse-led change and development, PhD thesis. Steinberg Collection, Royal College of Nursing, London.

Bellman L (2000) The surgical nurse as independent and collaborative practitioner. In Manley K and Bellman L (eds.) Surgical Nursing: Advancing Practice. Edinburgh: Churchill Livingstone .

Bellman L (2001) Courage, Faith and Chocolate Cake: requisites for exploring professionalism in action. Educational Action Research 9(2), 225-241.

Benner P (1984) From Novice to Expert - excellence and power in clinical nursing practice. California: Addison-Wesley.

Bennett R L, Baumann T and Battenhorst R L (1982) Morphine titration in postoperative laporotomy patients using patient-controlled analgesia. Current Therapeutic Research 32, 45-52.

Bennis W G, Benne K D and Chinn R (1985) The Planning of Change (fourth edition) Jovanovich, Fort Worth: Harcourt, Brace.

Berg B L (1989) Qualitative Research Methods for the Social sciences. New York: Allyn and Bacon.

Bertinasco L G (1990) Strategies for resolving conflict. Health Care Supervisor 8(4), 35-39.

Biley F (1989) Nurses' perceptions of stress in preoperative surgical patients. Journal of Advanced Nursing 14, 575-581.

Biley F (1991) The divide between theory and practice. Nursing 4(12), 28 February-13 March.

Bird C and Hassall J (1993) Self-Administration of Drugs. London: Scutari.

Boore J R P (1978) Prescription For Recovery. London: Royal College of Nursing.

Boud D, Keogh R and Walker D (eds.) (1985) Turning Experience into Learning. London: Kogan Page.

Bourdieu P (1977) Outline of a Theory of Practice. Cambridge: Cambridge University Press.

Bower F L (1977) The Process Of Planning Nursing Care: A Model For Practice. St Louis: Mosby.

Bowman G (1997) Over-managed. Nursing Standard 11, 19.

Boyatzis R E (1998) Transforming Qualitative Information: thematic analysis and code development. Thousand Oaks: SAGE.

Brechin A (2000) Introducing critical practice. In Brechin A, Brown H and Eby M A (eds.) Critical Practice in Health and Social Care. London: SAGE/Open University.

British Association of Medical Managers (1996) Principles into Practice: the involvement of clinical staff in the management of NHS trusts. Cheshire: British Association of Medical Managers.

Brooking J (1986) Patient and Family Participation in nursing care: the development of a nursing process measuring scale, PhD thesis. University of London, King's College.

Brooking J (1988) A scale to measure use of the nursing process. Nursing Times 85(15).

Burke W (1998) The interview. Nursing Management 4(8), 14-17.

Burrows D E (1997) Facilitation: a concept analysis. Journal of Advanced Nursing 25, 396-404.

Caine C and Kenrick M (1997) The role of clinical directorate managers in facilitating evidence-based practice: a report of an exploratory study. Journal of Nursing Management 5, 157-165.

Cameron-Buccheri R and Ogier M E (1994) The USA's nurse managers and UK's ward sisters: critical roles for empowerment. Journal of Clinical Nursing 3, 205-212.

Camiah S (1997) Utilisation of nursing research in practice and application strategies to raise research awareness amongst nurse practitioners; a model for success. Journal of Advanced Nursing 26, 1193-1202.

Carper B A (1978) Fundamental patterns of knowing. Advances in Nursing Science 1(1), 13-23.

Carr W and Kemmis S (1986) Being Critical: education, knowledge and action research. London: Falmer Press.

Carrington S (1993) Quality assurance in day surgery. Journal of One Day Surgery (January).

Cartwright D (ed.) (1963) Field Theory in Social Science: selected theoretical papers by Kurt Lewin. London: Tavistock Publications.

Casey N and Smith R (1997) Bringing nurses and doctors closer together. British Medical Journal 314, 617-618.

Cavanagh S (1992) Job satisfaction of nursing staff working in hospital. Journal of Advanced Nursing 17, 704-711.

Cavanagh S (1996) Mergers and acquisitions: some implications of cultural change. Journal of Nursing Management 4, 45-50.

CCHS (1991) Just for the Day: Children admitted to hospital for day treatment. London: CCHS.

Chang B L, Uman G C, Linn L, Ware J E and Kane R J (1994) Effect of systematically verifying components of nursing care on satisfaction in elderly ambulatory women. Western Journal of Nursing Research 6, 367-386.

Chinn P L and Kramer M K (1991) Theory and Nursing, a systematic approach (third edition). St Louis: Mosby.

Clark J (1982) Development of models and theories on the concept of nursing. Journal of Advanced Nursing 14, 762-775.

Clarke E, Dudley P, Edwards A, Rowland S, Ryan C and Winter R (1993) Ways of presenting and critiquing action research reports. Educational Action Research 1(3), 490-492.

Coeling H V and Wilcox J R (1994) Steps to collaboration. Nursing Administration Quarterly 18(4), 44-55.

Coffey A and Atkinson P (1996) Making Sense of Qualitative Data. Thousand Oaks: SAGE.

Coghlan D and Brannick T (2001) Doing Action Research in Your Own Organisation. London: SAGE.

Cohen L and Manion L (1984) Action Research. In Bell J et al. (eds.) Conducting Small-scale Investigations in Educational Management. London: Paul Chapman in association with the Open University.

Colaizzi P (1978) Psychological research as the phenomenologist views it. In Valle S and King M (eds.) Existential-phenomenological Alternatives for Psychology. Oxford: Oxford University Press.

Conway J (1996) Nursing Expertise and Advanced Practice. Dinton: Quay books.

Cope D E (1981) Organisational Development and Action Research in Hospitals. London: Gower.

Cormack D and Reynolds R (1992) Criteria for evaluating the clinical and practical utility of models used by nurses. Journal of Advanced Nursing 17, 1472-1478.

Cottrell N (1990) The view from the pharmacy. Nursing Times 86(43) (24 October).

Cowen S (1986) Care plan for a woman with an ectopic pregnancy based on Roper's activities of living model. In Webb C (ed.) Women's Health. London: Hodder and Stoughton.

Cox H, Hickson P and Taylor B (1991) Exploring reflection: knowing and constructing practice. In Gray G and Pratt R (eds.) Towards a Discipline of Nursing. Melbourne: Churchill Livingstone.

Crane S (1991) Implications of the critical paradigm. In Gray G and Pratt R (eds.) Towards a Discipline of Nursing. Melbourne: Churchill Livingstone.

Dadds M (1998) Supporting Practitioner Research: a challenge. Educational Action Research 6(1), 39-52.

Davidhizar R E (1994) Using facilitation as a managerial technique. Journal of Nursing Management 2, 193-196.

Davies S (1997) Research and development: How nurses can take a central role. NTresearch 2(1), 28-30.

Davis S (1991) Self-administration of medicines. Nursing Standard 5(15), 29-31 (9 January).

Daws J (1988) An inquiry into the attitudes of qualified nursing staff towards the use of nursing care plans. Journal of Advanced Nursing 13(1), 139-146.

D'Crutz J and Bottoff J (1984) Towards inclusive notions of patient and nurse. Journal of Advanced Nursing 9, 549-553.

DeMeester D W, Lauer T, Neal S E and Williams S (1989) Virginia Henderson: Definition of Nursing. In Marriner-Tomey A (ed.) Nursing Theorists and Their Work (second edition). St Louis: Mosby.

Denzin N K (1978) The Research Act: A Theoretical Introduction to Sociological Methods. New York: McGraw-Hill.

Department of Health (1986) Report of the Nursing Process Group to the DHSS. Nursing Research Liaison Group DHSS (May).

Department of Health (1989) Working for Patients: Caring for the 1990s, presented to Parliament by the Secretaries of State for Health, Wales, Northern Ireland, Scotland by command of Her Majesty. London: HMSO.

Department of Health (1991a) Research for Health: A Research and Development Strategy for the NHS. London: HMSO.

Department of Health (1991b) Welfare of Children and Young People in Hospital. London: HMSO.

Department of Health (1997) The New NHS - Modern, Dependable. London: HMSO.

Department of Health (1998) A First-class Service Quality in the new NHS, London: Department of Health.

Department of Health (1999) Making a Difference: strengthening the nursing, midwifery and health visiting contribution to health and healthcare. London: Department of Health.

Department of Health (2001) Shifting the Balance of Power within the NHS. London: Department of Health.

Department of Social Security (1987) Promoting Better Health. The Government's programme for improving primary healthcare. London: HMSO.

Dimond B (1995) UKCC's standards for incorporation into contracts. British Journal of Nursing 4(18), 1045-1046.

Dossey B M, and Keegan L (1988) Holistic Nursing: A Handbook For Practice. Rockville: Aspen.

Duffy K, and Scott PA (1998) Viewing an old issue through a new lens: a critical theory insight into the education-practice gap. Nurse Education Today 18, 183-189.

Dunham J and Fisher E (1990) Nurse executive profile of excellent nursing leadership. Nursing Administration Quarterly 15(1), 1-8.

East L and Robinson J (1993) Attitude Problem. Nursing Times 89(48), 1 December.

East L and Robinson J (1994) Change in process: bringing about change in healthcare through action research. Journal of Clinical Nursing 3, 57-61.

Eby M (2000) Understanding Professional Development. In Brechin A, Brown H and Eby M A (eds.) Critical Practice in Health and Social Care. London: SAGE/Open University.

Edmonstone J (1995) Managing change: an emerging new consensus. Health Manpower Management 21(1), 16-19.

Edmonstone J (2000) Empowerment in the national health service: does shared governance offer a way forward? Journal of Nursing Management 8, 259-264.

Elliott J (1978) What is action research in schools? Journal of Curriculum Studies 10, 355-357.

Elliott M and Turrell A (1996) Understanding the conflicts of patient empowerment. Nursing Standard 10(45), 43-47.

Ewles L and Simnett I (1992) Promoting Health. A Practical Guide (second edition). London: Scutari.

Ewles L and Simnett I (1999) Promoting Health. A Practical Guide (fourth edition). London: Scutari.

Farmer B (1993) The use and abuse of power in nursing. Nursing Standard 7(23), 33-36.

Farnish S (1983) Ward Sister Preparation: A Survey of Three Districts. Nursing Education Research Unit. Report No. 2, Chelsea College, University of London.

Faugier J (1992) Tall Poppies. Nursing Times 88(50), 20 (9 December).

Fawcett J (1989) Analysis and Evaluation of Conceptual Models of Nursing (second edition). Philadelphia: FA Davis.

Fay B (1987) Critical Social Science: Liberation and Limits. Cambridge: Polity Press.

Field P A and Morse J M (1985) Nursing Research: The Application of Qualitative Approaches. London: Chapman and Hall.

FitzGerald M (1995) The practical implications of a critique of traditional science. International Journal of Nursing Practice 1, 2-11.

Fitzpatrick J (1997) The power of politics and partnerships. Applied Nursing Research 10(4), 167.

Fitzpatrick R and Hopkins A (1983) Problems in the conceptual framework of patient satisfaction research. Sociology of Health and Illness 5, 297-311.

Fleming V E M and Moloney J A (1996) Critical social theory as grounded process. International Journal of Nursing Practice 2, 118-121.

Foale H (1991) Concerns in surgical paediatric nursing. Paediatric Nursing (February).

Forester J (1983) Critical Theory and Organisational Analysis. In Morgan G (ed.) Beyond Method. SAGE: Newbury Park.

Fraser M (1990) Using Conceptual Nursing Models in Practice - a research-based approach. London: Chapman and Hall.

Freidson E (1988) Profession of Medicine. A study of sociology applied knowledge. London: University of Chicago Press.

Fretwell J E (1982) Ward Teaching and Learning. London: Royal College of Nursing.

Fretwell J E (1985) Freedom to Change. The creation of a ward learning environment. London: Royal College of Nursing.

Frissell S (1988) So many models, so much confusion. Nursing Administration Quarterly 12(2), 13-17.

Fry A, Mortimor K and Ramsey L (1994) Clinical research and the culture of collaboration. The Australian Journal of Advanced Nursing 11(3), March-May.

Fulton Y (1997) Nurses' views on empowerment: a critical social theory perspective. Journal of Advanced Nursing 26, 529-536.

Gibson C (1991) A concept analysis of empowerment. Journal of Advanced Nursing 16, 354-361.

Giddens A (1985) Jurgen Habermas. In Skinner Q (ed.) The Return of the Grand Theory in the Human Sciences. Cambridge: Cambridge University Press.

Gilbert T (1995) Nursing: empowerment and the problem of power. Journal of Advanced Nursing 21, 865-871.

Gillis L (1988) Human Behaviour in Illness. London: Faber and Faber.

Girot E (1990) Discussing nursing theory. Senior Nurse 10(6), 16-19 June.

Goffman I (1961) Asylums. Penguin, Harmondsworth.

Goodman J (1989) Reflection and teacher education: a case study and theoretical analysis. Interchange 15(3), 9-26.

Grant G, Nolan M, Maguire B and Melhuish E (1994) Factors influencing job satisfaction among nurses. British Journal of Nursing 3(12), 615-620.

Greenwood J (1994) Action Research: a few details, a caution and something new. Journal of Advanced Nursing 20, 13-18.

Greenwood J (1995) Scholarship in Nursing Practice. In Gray G and Pratt R (eds.) Scholarship in the Discipline of Nursing. Melbourne: Churchill Livingstone.

Greenwood A (1997) Leadership for change. Nursing Standard 11(19), 22-24.

Grossman M and Hooton M (1993) The significance of the relationship between a discipline and its practice. Journal of Advanced Nursing 18, 866-872.

Grundy S (1982) Three modes of action research. Curriculum Perspectives 2(3), 23-34.

Gueldner S H and Stroud S D (1996) Sharing the quest for knowledge through interdisciplinary research. Holistic Nursing Practice 10(3), 54-62.

Guild of Hospital Pharmacists (1990) Self-medication systems. The Pharmaceutical Journal 28-29 (8 December).

Gunning R (1968) The Technique of Clear Writing. Philadelphia: McGraw Hill.

Habermas J (1972) Knowledge and Human Interests (trans. Shapiro J J). London: Heinemann.

Habermas J (1974) Theory and Practice (trans. Viertel J). London: Heinemann.

Habermas J (1976) Legitimation Crisis. London: Heinemann.

Habermas J (1979) Communication and the Evolution of Society (trans. McCarthy T). Boston, New England: Beacon Press.

Hagell E (1989) Nursing knowledge; women's knowledge: a sociological perspective. Journal of Advanced Nursing 14, 226-233.

Hamilton-Hurren A (1997) Empowerment. Nursing in Critical Care 2(3), 109-110.

Hammersley M (1992) What's wrong with Ethnography? London: Routledge.

Handy C (1985) On Power And Influence In Understanding Organisations. London: Penguin.

Hanson E J (1994) Issues concerning the familiarity of researchers within the research setting. Journal of Advanced Nursing 20(5), 940-942.

Harden J (1996) Enlightenment, empowerment and emancipation: the case for critical pedagogy in education. Nurse Education Today 16, 32-37.

Hart E (1995) Case study 2 - From sister to manager - empowerment through a staff development programme. In Hart E and Bond M, Action Research for Health and Social Care. London: Open University.

Hart E and Bond M (1995a) Developing action research in nursing. Nurse Researcher 2(3), 4-14.

Hart E and Bond M (1995b) Action Research for Health and Social Care. Buckingham: Open University Press.

Hart E and Bond M (1996) Making sense of action research through the use of typology. Journal of Advanced Nursing 23, 152-159.

Hawks J (1991) Power: a concept analysis. Journal of Advanced Nursing 16, 754-762.

Hayes P (1996) Is there a place for action research? Clinical Nursing Research 5(1), 3-4.

Hayward J (1975) Information: A Prescription Against Pain. London: Royal College of Nursing.

Hayward A J, Will V E, MacAskill S and Hastings G B (1991) Retention Within the Nursing Profession in Scotland, University of Strathclyde, Glasgow.

Health Education Authority (1990) Promoting Better Health and the GP Contract. London: Health Education Authority.

Hendricks-Thomas J and Patterson E (1995) A sharing in critical thought by nursing faculty. Journal of Advanced Nursing 22, 594-599.

Hendry C and Farley A H (1996) The nurse teacher as Action Researcher. Nurse Education Today 16, 193-198.

Henneman E A, Lee J L and Cohen J I (1995) Collaboration: a concept analysis. Journal of Advanced Nursing 21, 103-109.

Heslop L (1997) The (im)possibilities of post-structuralist and critical social nursing inquiry. Nursing Inquiry 4, 48-56.

Hickey J V, Ouimette R M and Venegoni S L (eds.) (1996) Advanced Practice Nursing: changing roles and clinical applications,. Philadelphia: Lippincott.

Hirschfeld M J (1998) WHO priorities for a common nursing research agenda. Image: Journal of Nursing Scholarship 30(2), 114.

Holloway I (1992) Patients as participants in research. Senior Nurse 12(3), 46-47.

Holloway G and Race A J (1993) Developing a rationale for research-based practice: some considerations for nurse teachers. Nurse Education Today 13, 259-263.

Holmes C (1996) Resistance to positivist science in nursing: an assessment of the Australian literature. International Journal of Nursing Practice 2, 172-181.

Holter I M and Schwartz-Barcott D (1993) Action Research: what is it? How has it been used and how can it be used in nursing? Journal of Advanced Nursing 18, 298-304.

Huckabay L (1991) The role of conceptual frameworks in nursing practice, administration, education and research. Nursing Administration Quarterly 15(3), 17-28 (winter).

Hugentobler M K, Israel B A and Schurman S J (1992) An action research approach to workplace health: integrating methods. Health Education Quarterly 19(1), 55-76.

Huntington A, Gilmour J and O'Connell A (1996) Reforming the practice of nurses: decolonization or getting out from under. Journal of Advanced Nursing 24, 364-367.

Huxham C (ed.) (1996) Creating Collaborative Advantage. London: SAGE.

Iles V (1997) Really Managing Health Care. Buckingham: Open University Press.

Iles V and Sutherland K (2001) Organisational Change: a review for healthcare managers, professionals and researchers. National Co-ordinating Centre for NHS Service Delivery and Organisation R&D. London: NCCSDO.

Ingram R (1991) Why does nursing need theory? Journal of Advanced Nursing 16, 350-353.

James C J (1993) Developing reflective practice skills - the potential. Paper presented to the 'Power of the Portfolio' national conference, Nottingham, 12 November.

Jick T D (1983) Mixing qualitative methods: triangulation in action. In Vans Maanen J (ed.) Qualitative Methodology. Beverley Hills, California: SAGE.

Johns C (1993) Professional supervision. Journal of Nursing Management 1(1).

Johnson M (1997a) Observations on the neglected concept of intervention in nursing research. Journal of Advanced Nursing 5, 23-29.

Johnson M (1997b) Nursing Power and Social Judgement. Aldershot: Ashgate.

Johnson M B (1990) The holistic paradigm in nursing: the diffusion of an innovation Research in Nursing and Health 13, 129-139.

Johnson G and Scholes K (1993) Exploring Corporate Strategy-Text and Cases (third edition). London: Prentice Hall.

Jones W (1996) Triangulation in clinical practice. Journal of Clinical Nursing 5, 319-323.

Jones M (1997) Thinking nursing. In Thorne S E and Hayes V (eds.) Nursing Praxis: knowledge and action. Thousand Oaks: SAGE.

Jukes M (1988) Nursing model or psychological assessment. Senior Nurse 8(1).

Kemmis S (1981) Research approaches and methods: action research. In Anderson A and Blackers C (eds.) Transition From School: an exploration of research and policy. Canberra: Australian National University Press.

Kemmis S (1985) Action research and the politics of reflection. In Boud D, Keogh R and Walker D (eds.) Reflection, Turning Experience into Learning. London: Kogan Page.

Kenny T (1993) Nursing models fail in practice. British Journal of Nursing 2(2), 133-136.

Kershaw B (1992) Models of Nursing in Jolley M and Brykczynka G (eds.) Nursing Care - the challenge to change. London: Edward Arnold.

Keyzer D (1985) Using learning contracts to support change in nursing organisations. Nurse Education Today 6(3), 103-108.

Kilgour D Y and Logan W W (1985) A model for health: its use in an undergraduate nursing programme. Nurse Education Today 5(5), 215-220.

Kim H S and Holter I M (1995a) Critical theory for science of nursing practice. In Omery A, Kasper C E and Page G G (eds.) In Search of Nursing Science. London: SAGE.

Kim H S and Holter I M (1995b) Methodology for critical theory. In Omery A, Kasper C E and Page G G (eds.) In Search of Nursing Science. London: SAGE.

Kincheloe J L and McLaren P L (1994) Rethinking critical theory and qualitative research. In Denzin N K and Lincoln Y S (eds.) Handbook of Qualitative Research. London: SAGE.

King's Fund (1991) Organisational Audit. London: King Edward's Hospital Fund.

Klakovich M D (1994) Connective leadership for the 21st century: a historical perspective and future directions. Advances in Nursing Science 16(4), 42-54.

Kolb D A (1984) Experiential Learning. New Jersey: Prentice Hall.

Krouse J K and Roberts S J (1989) Nurse-patient interactive styles: power, control, satisfaction. Western Journal of Nursing Research 11(6), 717-725.

Kubler-Ross E (1969) On Death and Dying. New York: Macmillan.

Lancaster J (1999) Nursing Issues in Leading and Managing Change. St Louis: Mosby.

Lancaster J and Lancaster W (eds.) (1982) The Nurse as a Change Agent. St Louis: Mosby.

Lather P (1991) Getting Smart. London: Routledge.

Lathlean J and Farnish S (1984) The Ward Sister Training Project: An Evaluation of a Training Scheme. Nursing Education Research Unit. Report No. 3. London: Chelsea College, University of London.

Le May A, Alexander C and Mulhall A (1998) Research-based practice: practitioners' and managers' views. Managing Clinical Nursing 2, 87-92.

Leenders F (1996) An overview of policies guiding healthcare for children. Nursing Standard 10(28), 33-38.

Lenkman S and Gribbins R (1994) Multidisciplinary teams in the acute care setting. Holistic Nurse Practice 8(3), 81-87.

Lewin K (1947) Group decision and social change. In Maccoby E E, Newcomb T M and Hartley E L (eds.) Readings in Social Psychology. New York: Holt, Rinehart and Winston.

Lewin K (1952) Field Theory in Social Science. London: Tavistock.

Lewin K, Dembo I, Festinger L and Sears P S (1944) Levels of Aspiration. In Hunt J (ed.) Personality and Behaviour Disorder: a handbook based on experimental and clinical research. New York: The Ronald Press.

Lister P E (1991) Approaching models of nursing from a postmodernist perspective. Journal of Advanced Nursing 16, 206-212.

Lofland J and Lofland L H (1984) Analyzing Social Settings. A Guide to Qualitative Observation and Analysis. Belmont, California: Wadsworth.

Long R (1981) Systematic Nursing Care. London: Faber and Faber.

Lont K (1995) Critical theory scholarship and nursing. In Gray G and Pratt R (eds.) Scholarship in the Discipline of Nursing. Melbourne: Churchill Livingstone.

Lorentzon M (1993) Research for health; managing the nursing input. Journal of Nursing Management 1, 39-46.

Lucock R (1997) Action Research: dissertation appendix (MSc) in Nursing (distance learning) study guide. London: Royal College of Nursing.

Lumby J (1996) Stressors in the life of the contemporary nurse. International Journal of Nursing Practice 2, 45-46.

McCaughtery D (1992) The Roper nursing model as an educational research tool. British Journal of Nursing 1(9), 455-459.

McConnell C (1995) Delegation versus empowerment: what, how and is there a difference? Health Care Supervisor 14, 69-79.

McKenna H (1989) The selection by ward managers of an appropriate nursing model for long-stay psychiatric care. Journal of Advanced Nursing 14, 762-775.

Mackenzie J (1993) Effects of change on sisters/charge nurses. Nursing Standard 7(36), 25-27.

McKernan J (1996) Curriculum Action Research (second edition). London: Kogan Page.

McNiff J (1988) Action Research Principles and Practice. Basingstoke: Macmillan Education Limited.

McNiff J, Lomax P and Whitehead J (1996) You and Your Action Research Project. London: Routledge.

McTaggart R (1982) The Action Research Planner. Deakin University Press, Victoria, Australia.

Maggs-Rapport F (2001) 'Best Research Practice': in pursuit of methodological rigour. Journal of Advanced Nursing 35(3), 373-383.

Malby R (1997) Developing the future leaders of nursing in the UK. European Nurse 2(1), 27-36.

Malin N and Teasdale K (1991) Caring versus empowerment: considerations for nursing practice. Journal of Advanced Nursing 16, 657-662.

Manley K (1997) A conceptual framework for advanced practice: an action research project operationalizing an advanced practitioner/consultant nurse role. Journal of Clinical Nursing 6(3), 179-190.

Manley K and Bellman L (2000) Surgical Nursing: Advancing Practice. Edinburgh: Churchill Livingstone.

Manley K and McCormack B (1997) Exploring Expert Practice. MSc. in Nursing Distance Learning Study Guide. London: Royal College of Nursing.

Marson SN (1982) Ward sister-teacher or facilitator? An investigation into the behavioural characteristics of effective ward teachers. Journal of Advanced Nursing 7, 347-357.

Maslin-Prothero S and Masterson A (1998) Continuing care: developing a policy analysis for nursing. Journal of Advanced Nursing 28(3), 548-553.

Maslow A H (1954) Motivation and Personality. New York: Harper and Row.

Masterson A (1993) Concept analysis of independence. Surgical Nurse 6(6), 27-29 December.

May C (1998) The preparation and analysis of qualitative interview data. In Roe B and Webb C (eds.) Research and Development in Clinical Nursing Practice. London: Whurr.

Meleis A I (1997) Theoretical Nursing: Development and Progress (third edition). Philadelphia: Lippincott.

Meleis A I and Burton P S (1981) Innovative educational changes: a paradigm. International Journal of Nursing Studies 18, 33-39.

Meyer J (1993a) New paradigm research: the trials and tribulations of action research. Journal of Advanced Nursing 18, 1066-1072.

Meyer J (1993b) Lay participation in care: a challenge for multidisciplinary team-work. Journal of Interprofessional Care 7(1), 57-66.

Meyer J (1995) Stages in the process: a personal account. Nurse Researcher 2(3), 24-37.

Meyer J (2001) Action Research. In Fulop N, Allen P, Clarke A and Black N (eds.) Studying the Organisation and Delivery of Health Services. London: Routledge.

Meyer J and Bateup L (1997) Action research in health-care practice: nature: present concerns and future possibilities. NTresearch 2(3), 175-184.

Mezirow J (1981) A critical theory of adult learning and education. Adult Education 32(3), 3-24.

Miles M B and Huberman A M (1984) Qualitative Data Analysis. A Source Book of New Methods. Newbury Park, California: SAGE.

Minardi H A and Riley M (1988) Providing psychological safety through skilled communication. Nursing 27, 990-992.

Minor J (1998) Can we really blow the whistle? Nursing Management 5(3), 11-14.

Minshull J and Ross K (1986) The human needs model of nursing. Journal of Advanced Nursing 11, 643-649.

Mitchell J R A (1984) Is nursing any business of doctors? A simple guide to the 'nursing process'. British Medical Journal 288, 216-219.

Moore S (1990) Thoughts on the discipline of nursing as we approach the year 2000. Journal of Advanced Nursing 15, 825-828.

Morgan M and Reynolds A (1991) Day surgery units: are they attractive to nurses? Journal of Advances in Health and Nursing Care 1(2), 59-74.

Morton N S (1993) Paediatric day case anaesthesia. The Journal of One Day Surgery, Autumn, 22.

Morton-Cooper A (2000) Action Research in Health Care. Oxford: Blackwell Science Ltd.

Mulhall A and le May (2001) Taking action. Moving towards evidence-based practice. London: The Foundation of Nursing Studies.

National Association of Theatre Nurses (1996) Nursing the Paediatric Patient in the Adult Peri-operative Environment. Harrogate: National Association of Theatre Nurses.

Newton C (1991) The Roper, Logan and Tierney Model in Action. Basingstoke: Macmillan.

Nicholl S, King T A and Knowles L (1996) Adapting an adult day surgery unit for paediatric work. The Journal of One Day Surgery 10-11, Spring.

Nolan M and Grant G (1993) Action research and quality of care: a mechanism for agreeing basic values as a precursor to change. Journal of Advanced Nursing 18, 305-311.

Nuffield Hospitals (1994) Setting standards for children undergoing surgery. London: Action for Sick Children, Nuffield Hospitals.

O'Connor A M (1997) Consumer/patient decision support in the new millenium: where should our research take us? Canadian Journal of Nursing Research 29(3), 7-12.

O'Kelly G (1994) Empowerment of the nurse. Nursing Review 13(1), 13-15.

Ogier M E (1982) An Ideal Sister? London: Royal College of Nursing.

Ogier M E (1986) An ideal sister - seventy years on? Nursing Times. Occasional paper 82, vol. 2, 54-57.

Ogier M E (1989) Working and Learning. London: Scutari.

Oja S N and Smulyan L (1989) Collaborative Action Research. London: Falmer Press.

Olsen E M (1979) Strategies and techniques for the nurse change agent. Nursing Clinics of North America 14, 323-336.

Orton H D (1981) Ward Learning Climate. London: Royal College of Nursing.

Ovretveit J (1997) How patient power and client participation affects relations between professions. In Ovretveit J, Mathias P and Thompson T (eds.) Interprofessional Working for Health and Social Care. London: Macmillan.

Owen H, Mather L and Rowley K (1988) The development and clinical use of patient-controlled analgesia. Anaesthesia and Intensive Care 16(4), 437-447.

Owen-Mills V (1995) A synthesis of caring praxis and critical theory in an emancipatory curriculum. Journal of Advanced Nursing 21, 1191-1195.

Parker D (1997) Nursing art and science: literature and debate. In Marks-Maran D and Rose P (eds.) Reconstructing Nursing: Beyond Art and Science. London: Baillière Tindall.

Parrott T E (1994) Humour as a teaching strategy. Nurse Educator 19(3), May/June.

Parsloe P (1997) Everyday choices may be as important as the 'grand notion'. Care Plan 3(3), 9-12. Anglia Polytechnic University.

Parsons T (1951) The Social System. New York: Free Press.

Patronis Jones R A (1994) Conceptual development of nurse-physician collaboration. Holistic Nurse Practice 8(3), 1-11.

Patton M Q (1990) Qualitative Evaluation and Research Methods (second edition). Newbury Park, California: SAGE.

Pearson A and Vaughan B (1986) Nursing Models for Practice. London: Heinemann.

Pembery S (1980) The Ward Sister - Key to Nursing. London: Royal College of Nursing.

Peters M, and Robinson V (1984) The origins and status of action research. The Journal of Applied Behavioural Science 20(2), 113-124.

Phippen M L (1980) Nursing assessment of preoperative anxiety. Association of Operating Rooms. Nurses Journal 31(6), 1019-1026.

Plowes D and Fudge L (2000) Perspectives on major disaster nursing in the developing world. In Manley K and Bellman L (eds.) Surgical Nursing: Advancing Practice. Edinburgh: Churchill Livingstone.

Polit D F and Hungler B P (1985) Essentials of Nursing Research Methods and Applications. Philadelphia: Lippincott.

Porter R (1997) The Greatest Benefit to Mankind. London: Harper Collins.

Powell J H (1989) The reflective practitioner in nursing. Journal of Advanced Nursing 14, 824-832.

Powers B A (1995) A Dictionary of Nursing Theory and Research. Newbury Park, California: SAGE.

Powers B A and Knapp T R (1990) A Dictionary of Nursing Theory and Research. Newbury Park, California: SAGE.

Pryjmachuk S (1996) Pragmatism and change: some implications for nurses, nurse managers and nursing. Journal of Nursing Management 4, 201-205.

Quinn S (1989) Work with Nurses: a profession in transition. In Klein L (ed.) Working With Organisations. Loxwood: Kestral.

Rabinow P (ed.) (1991) The Foucault Reader. London: Penguin.

Raelin J (1989) An anatomy of autonomy: managing professionals. Academy of Management Executives 3(3), 216-227.

Rasmussen S (1997) Action research as authentic methodology for the study of nursing. In Thorne S E and Hayes V E (eds.) Nursing Praxis: knowledge and action. Thousand Oaks: SAGE.

Ray M A (1992) Critical theory as a framework to enhance nursing science. Nursing Science Quarterly 5(3), 98-100.

Reason P (1995) Participation: consciousness and constitutions. Paper prepared for the American Academy of Management Conference, May 3-6, University of Bath.

Reason P and Marshall J (1987) Research as personal process. In Boud D and Griffin V (eds.) Appreciating Adults Learning: From the Learners' Perspective. London: Kogan Page.

Reed J (1992) Secondary data in nursing research. Journal of Advanced Nursing 17, 877-883.

Reed G (1995) A treatise on nursing knowledge development for the 21st century: beyond postmodernism. Advances in Nursing Science 17(3), 70-84.

Reed J and Procter S (1993) Nurse education: a reflective approach. London: Edward Arnold.

Reed J and Robbins I (1991) Models of Nursing: their relevance to the care of elderly people. Journal of Advanced Nursing 16, 1350-1357.

Reports (1996) Taking on junior doctors' roles: who is accountable? Nursing Standard 10(39), 32 (19 June).

Retsas A (1994) Knowledge and practice development: toward an ontology of nursing. The Australian Journal of Advanced Nursing 12(2), 20-25.

Riley J (1990) Getting The Most From Your Data. A handbook of practical ideas on how to analyse qualitative data. Bristol: Technical and Educational Services Limited.

Riley J M and Omery A (1996) The scholarship of a practice discipline. Holistic Nursing Practice 10(3), 7-14.

Roberts S J (1983) Oppressed group behaviour: implications for nursing. Advances in Nursing Science (21-30 July).

Roberts S J (1997) Nurse Executives in the 1990s: empowered or oppressed? Nurse Administration Quaterly 22(1), 64-71.

Robinson D (1989) Response rates in questionnaires. Senior Nurse 9(10), 25-26.

Robinson K (1990) Nursing Models - the hidden costs. Surgical Nurse 3(1), 11-14.

Robinson J (1997) Power, Politics and Policy Analysis in nursing. In Perry A (ed.) Nursing: A Knowledge Base for Practice. London: Edward Arnold.

Rodwell C M (1996) An analysis of the concept of empowerment. Journal of Advanced Nursing 23, 305-313.

Roediger H L, Rushton J P, Capaldi E D and Paris S G (1987) Psychology. Toronto: Little, Brown International Student Edition.

Rogers E (1962) The Diffusion of Innovations. New York: Free Press.

Rogers E M (1989) Creating a climate for the implementation of a nursing conceptual framework. Journal of Continuing Education in Nursing 20(3), 112-116.

Rogers E M (1995) Diffusion of Innovations (fourth edition). New York: Free Press.

Rolfe G (1994) Towards a new model of nursing research. Journal of Advanced Nursing 19, 969-975.

Rolfe G (1998) Expanding Nursing Knowledge. Oxford: Butterworth Heinemann UK.

Roper N (1976) Clinical Experience in Nurse Education. Edinburgh: Churchill Livingstone.

Roper N (2000) Roper, Logan and Tierney Model of Nursing: based on activities of living. Edinburgh: Churchill Livingstone.

Roper N and Logan W (1983) Using a model for nursing. Edinburgh: Churchill Livingstone.

Roper N and Logan W (1985) The Roper, Logan and Tierney model. Senior Nurse 3(2), 20-26, July.

Roper N, Logan W and Tierney A (1980) The Elements of Nursing. Edinburgh: Churchill Livingstone.

Roper N, Logan W and Tierney A (1981) Learning to Use the Process of Nursing. Edinburgh: Churchill Livingstone.

Roper N, Logan W and Tierney A (1990) The Elements of Nursing (third edition). Edinburgh: Churchill Livingstone.

Roper N, Logan W and Tierney A (1996) The Elements of Nursing: A Model for Nursing Based on a Model for Living (fourth edition). Edinburgh: Churchill Livingstone.

Royal College of Surgeons (1992) Guidelines for Day Case Surgery. London: Commission on the Provision of Surgical Services, Royal College of Surgeons of England.

Rubright P (1984) Persuading Physicians. Rockville: Aspen.

Runciman PJ (1983) Ward Sister at Work. Edinburgh: Churchill Livingstone.

Salvage J (1990) The theory and practice of the new nursing. Nursing Times 86(4), 24 January.

Sapsford R and Abbott P (1992) Research Methods for Nurses and the Caring Professions. Buckingham: Open University Press.

Schlotfeldt R M (1975) The need for a conceptual framework. In Verhonick J (ed.) Nursing Research. Boston, New England: Little, Brown and Company.

Schon D A (1983) The Reflective Practitioner. London: Temple Smith.

Schon D A (1991) The Reflective Practitioner (second edition). San Francisco: Jossey Bass.

Schrober J (1991) The Organisation of Care Module Handbook, Diploma in Nursing. Southbank University, London: Distance Learning Centre.

Schwartz D and Jacobs J (1979) Qualitative Sociology: A Method to the Madness. New York: Free Press.

Scriven L (1987) Self-medication in a surgical ward. New Zealand Nursing Journal 25-26, December.

Seabrook M (1998) Overcoming tribalism. Nursing Standard 12(20), 23-24.

Shea H M (1986) A conceptual framework to study the use of nursing care plans. International Journal of Nursing Studies 23(2), 147-157.

Shea H M, Rogers M, Ross E, Tucker D, Fitch M and Smith I (1989) Implementation of nursing conceptual models: observations of a multi-site research team. Canadian Journal of Nursing Administration 2 (1), 15-20.

Sheehan J (1986) Aspects of research methodology. Nurse Education Today 6, 193-203.

Shipman M (1988) The Limitations of Social Research (third edition) London: Longman.

Sills E (1993) The power struggle. Journal of Clinical Nursing 2(1), 4.

Silva M C (1986) Research testing nursing theory: state of the art. Advances in Nursing Science 9(1), 1-11.

Silva M C and Sorrell J M (1992) Testing of nursing theory: critique and philosophical expansion. Advances in Nursing Science 14(4), 12-23.

Simons H (2000) On what evidence do we act in developing and using professional knowledge? Reinterpreting Evidence-based Practice: A Narrative Approach. Collaborative Action Research Network/South Thames Postgraduate Medical and Dental Education, CARE, University of East Anglia.

Sines D (1994) The arrogance of power: a reflection on contemporary mental health nursing practice. Journal of Advanced Nursing 20, 894-903.

Skidmore D (1989) Flexibility: the key to success. Nursing Times 85(48), 52-53, 29 November.

Smith L (1990) A suitable case for intimacy. The Lancet 33(6), 217-218.

Smith M C (1990) Nursing practice: guided by or generating theory. Nursing Science Quarterly 3(4), 147-148 (Winter).

Smith J (1996) Empowering People. London: Kogan Page.

Smith R E, Ascough J C, Ettinger R F and Nelson DA (1971) Humour, anxiety and task performance. Journal Personality Social Psychology 19, 243-246.

Smyth W J (1987) A rationale for teacher's critical pedagogy: a handbook. Victoria, Australia: Deakin University Press.

Soltis-Jarrett V (1997) The facilitator in participatory action research: les raisons d'etre. Advances in Nursing Science 20(2), 45-54.

Speedy S (1989) Theory-practice debate: setting the scene. Australian Journal of Advanced Nursing 6(3), March-May.

Spiers C (2000) The surgical nurse as teacher and health promoter. In Manley K and Bellman L (2000) Surgical Nursing: Advancing Practice. Edinburgh: Churchill Livingstone.

Stein L, Watts D and Howell T (1990) Sounding Board; the nurse-doctor game revisited. New England Journal of Medicine 322(8), 548-549.

Stevens B J (1972) Why won't nurses write nursing care plans? Journal of Nursing Administation, November/December.

Stevens P E (1989) A critical social reconceptualisation of environment in nursing: implications for methodology. Advances in Nursing Science 11(4), 56-68.

Street A (1995) Nursing Replay. Melbourne: Churchill Livingstone.

Street A (1997) Thinking about nursing futures. Nursing Inquiry 4, 79.

Stringer E T (1999) Action Research: a Handbook for Practitioners. Thousand Oaks: SAGE.

Suominen T, Kovasin M and Ketola O (1997) Nursing culture - some viewpoints. Journal of Advanced Nursing 25(1), 186-190.

Suppe F and Jacox A K (1985) Philosophy of science and the development of nursing theory. In Werley H H and Fitzpatrick J J (eds.) Annual Review of Nursing Research. New York: Springer.

Surman L and Wright S (1998) Costs and Conflicts. In Wright S (ed.) Changing Nursing Practice (second edition). London: Arnold.

Susman G I and Evred R D (1978) An assessment of the scientific merits of action research. Administrative Science Quarterly 23, 583-601.

Sutton F and Smith C (1995) Advanced nursing practice: new idea and new perspectives. Journal of Advanced Nursing 21, 1037-1043.

Swan J and McVicar B (1992) The rough guide to change. Nursing Times 88(13), 48-49.

Sweet J and Norman I (1995) The nurse-doctor relationship: a selective literature review. Journal of Advanced Nursing 22, 165-170.

Tampoe M (1998) Liberating Leadership. London: The Industrial Society.

Taylor AG, Skelton JA and Czakowski J (1982) Do patients understand patient education brochures? Nursing and Health Care 3: 305–310.

Taylor B (1993) 'Ordinariness' in nursing: a study (part 2). Nursing Standard 7(40), 23 July.

Teasdale K (1993) Information and anxiety: a critical appraisal. Journal of Advanced Nursing 18, 1125-1132.

Thomas E (1992) Self-medication. Nursing 5 (2), 26-27.

Thomas N (1993) Patient and staff perceptions of patient PCA. Nursing Standard 7(28), 37–39.

Thomas V J and Rose F D (1993) Patient-controlled analgesia: a new method for old. Journal of Advanced Nursing 18, 1719-1726.

Thompson D R (1998) The art and science of research in clinical nursing. In Roe B and Webb C (eds.) Research and Development in Clinical Nursing Practice. London: Whurr.

Thompson I, Melia K and Boyd K (1988) Nursing Ethics. Edinburgh: Churchill Livingstone.

Thornes R (1991) Day admission for children. The Journal of One Day Surgery (June), 14.

Tierney A (1998) Nursing models: extant or extinct? Journal of Advanced Nursing 28(1), 77-85.

Tiffany C R and Lutjens L R J (1998) Planned Change Theories for Nursing. Thousand Oaks: SAGE.

Titchen A and Binnie A (1993) Changing power relationships between nurses: a case-study of early changes towards patient-centred nursing. Journal of Clinical Nursing 2, 219-229.

Torbert W R (1991) The Power of Balance: Transforming Self, Society and Social Inquiry. Newbury Park, California: SAGE.

Towell D (1996) Revaluing the NHS: empowering ourselves to shape a healthcare system fit for the 21st century. Policy and Politics 24(3), 287-297.

Towell D and Harries C (1979) Innovations in Patient Care. An Action Research Study of Change in a Psychiatric Hospital. London: Croom Helm.

Tross G and Cavanagh S J (1996) Innovation in nursing management: professional, management and methodological considerations. Journal of Nursing Management 4, 143-149.

Tuthill V (1995) The training of nurse surgical assistants. Surgical Nurse 4(21), 1240-1245.

United Kingdom Central Council (1990) Post-registration Education and Practice Project. London: UKCC.

United Kingdom Central Council (1997) (Scope in Practice). London: UKCC.

Uys L R (1987) Foundation studies in nursing. Journal of Advanced Nursing 12, 275-280.

Velianoff G D (1986) The nursing care plan as a teaching tool. Nursing Management (September).

Waite T (1997) Vocations. Nursing Standard 11(50), 16.

Walker P (2001) JAN Forum: Saving the discipline - Top 10 unfinished issues to inform the nursing debate in the new millenium. Journal of Advanced Nursing 35 (1), 138 (July).

Walker L O and Avant K C (1988) Strategies for Theory Construction in Nursing (second edition). Norwalk, Connecticut/San Mateo, California: Appleton and Lange.

Walsh M (1989) Model example. Nursing Standard 3, 23-25, 25 February.

Walsh M (1991) Models in Clinical Nursing: the way forward. London: Baillière Tindall.

Walsh M (1998) Models and Critical Pathways in Clinical Nursing. London: Baillière Tindall.

Walshe K (2000) Developing clinical governance: leadership, culture and change. Journal of Clinical Governance 8, 166-173.

Walshe K, Freeman T, Latham L, Spurgeon P and Wallace L (2000) Scope to Improve. Health Service Journal, 26 October.

Walton I (1986) The Nursing Process in Perspective: A Literature Review. University of York: Department of Social Policy and Social Work.

Warelow P J (1996) Nurse-doctor relationships in multidisciplinary teams: ideal or real? International Journal of Nursing Practice 2, 33-39.

Warelow P J (1997) A nursing journey through discursive praxis. Journal of Advanced Nursing 26, 1020-1027.

Waterman H (1995) Distinguishing between 'traditional' and action research. Nurse Researcher 2(3), 15-23.

Waterman H (1998) Embracing ambiguities and valuing ourselves: issues of validity in action research. Journal of Advanced Nursing 28(1), 101-105.

Waterman H, Webb C and Williams A (1995) Changing nursing and nursing change: a dialectical analysis of an action research project. Educational Action Research 3(1), 55-70.

Waterman H, Tillen D, Dickson R and de Koning K (2001) Action research: a systematic review and guidance for assessment. Health Technology Assessment 5, 23 (executive summary): www.ncchta.org/fullmono/mon523.pdf.

Watkins M (1993) Can you tread this emotional high wire? Professional Nurse (June), 604-608.

Watson-Druee N (1994) Grow your own staff. Nursing Management 1(2), 24-25 (May).

Webb C (1989) Action research, philosophy, methodology - personal experience. Journal of Advanced Nursing 14, 403-410.

Webb C (1991) Action Research. In Cormack DFS (ed.) The Reseach Process in Nursing (second edition). Oxford: Blackwell Science.

Webb C (1993) Action research: philosophy, methods and personal experience. In Kitson A (ed.) Nursing: Art and Science. London: Chapman and Hall.

Webb C (1996) Action research. In Cormack DFS (ed.) The Reseach Process in Nursing (second edition). Oxford: Blackwell Science.

Webster R (1990) The role of the nurse teacher. Senior Nurse 10(8), 16-18.

Weiss S J (1985) Role differentiation between nurses and physicians: implications for nursing. Nursing Research 32(3), 133-139.

Wheatley R and Smith C (1995) Leadership In Management Directions 3. Corby: The Institute of Management Foundation.

While A E and Wilcox V K (1994) Paediatric day surgery: day-case unit admission compared with general paediatric ward admission. Journal of Advanced Nursing 19, 52-57.

White P (1998) Fighting Nursing Management 4(8), 7.

White S K (ed.) (1988) The Cambridge Companion to Habermas. Cambridge: Cambridge University Press.

Williams A (1995) Ethics and action research. Nurse Researcher 2(3), 49-59.

Wilson J (1997) Introduction to integrated care management - introducing multidisciplinary pathways of care into an organisation through project, risk and change management. In Wilson J (ed.) Integrated Care Management: the Path to Success? London: Butterworth Heinemann UK.

Wilson-Thomas L (1995) Applying critical social theory in nursing education to bridge the gap between theory, research and practice. Journal of Advanced Nursing 21, 568-575.

Winter R (1989) Learning From Experience. Principles and Practice in Action Research. London: Falmer Press.

Wolcott H F (1994) Transforming Qualitative Data: description analysis and interpretation. Thousand Oaks: SAGE.

Woods L P (2000) The Enigma of Advanced Nursing Practice. Dinton: Quay Books.

World Health Organisation (1996) Nursing Practice. WHO Technical Report Series, no. 860. Switzerland:World Health Organisation.

Wright S (1986) Building and Using a Model of Nursing. London: Edward Arnold.

Wright S (1989) Changing Nursing Practice. London: Edward Arnold.

Wright S (1996) The need to develop nursing practice through innovation and practice change. International Journal of Nursing Practice 2, 142-148.

Wright S (ed.) (1998) Changing Nursing Practice (second edition) London: Edward Arnold.

Wright A, Brown P and Sloman R (1996) Nurses' perceptions of the value of nursing research for practice. Australian Journal of Advanced Nursing 13(4), 15-18.

Yuen F and Owens J (1996) Power in partnership. International Journal of Nursing Practice 2, 138-141.

Zuber-Skerritt O (1996) Emancipatory action research for organisational change and management development. In Zuber-Skerritt O (ed.) New Directions in Action Research. London: Falmer Press.

Index